# Dermatology - The Latest Research on Common Skin Diseases

*Edited by Shahin Aghaei*

Published in London, United Kingdom

Dermatology - The Latest Research on Common Skin Diseases
http://dx.doi.org/10.5772/intechopen.1004470
Edited by Shahin Aghaei

Contributors
Abhinav Vempati, Asma Damizadeh, Aya Mtiri, Crystal Zhou, Curtis Tam, Falk G. Bechara, Ghada Bouslama, Jeffrey Khong, Joshua Bronte, Lamia Oualha, Lennart Ocker, Lidiya Todorova, Nessr Abu Rached, Nour Sayda Ben Messaoud, Rawan Almutairi, Salar Hazany, Shahin Aghaei, Souha Ben Youssef, Taha Ashouritalouki

Notice

Statements and opinions expressed in the chapters are these of the individual contributors and not necessarily those of the editors or publisher. No responsibility is accepted for the accuracy of information contained in the published chapters. The publisher assumes no responsibility for any damage or injury to persons or property arising out of the use of any materials, instructions, methods or ideas contained in the book.

First published in London, United Kingdom, 2025 by IntechOpen
IntechOpen is the global imprint of INTECHOPEN LIMITED, registered in England and Wales, registration number: 11086078, 167-169 Great Portland Street, London, W1W 5PF, United Kingdom

For EU product safety concerns: IN TECH d.o.o., Prolaz Marije Krucifikse Kozulić 3, 51000 Rijeka, Croatia, info@intechopen.com or visit our website at intechopen.com.

British Library Cataloguing-in-Publication Data
A catalogue record for this book is available from the British Library

Dermatology - The Latest Research on Common Skin Diseases
Edited by Shahin Aghaei
p. cm.
Print ISBN 978-0-85014-900-5
Online ISBN 978-0-85014-899-2
eBook (PDF) ISBN 978-0-85014-901-2

If disposing of this product, please recycle the paper responsibly.

# IntechOpen

intechopen.com

## Built by scientists, for scientists

# Meet the editor

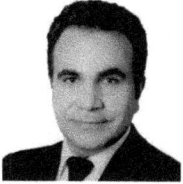

Shahin Aghaei, MD, graduated from Shiraz University of Medical Sciences, Shiraz, Iran, in 2004. He was awarded a fellowship in Dermatopathology by the International Society of Dermatology (ISD) from Charles University in Prague, Czech Republic, in 2008, and a fellowship in Dermatologic Surgery from the Medical University of Graz, Austria, in 2010. He is currently the editor-in-chief of the Journal of Surgical Dermatology in Singapore and an Associate Professor of Dermatology and Dermatologic Surgery at the Iran University of Medical Sciences School of Medicine, Tehran, Iran. He is also a member of the following medical societies: the American Academy of Dermatology, the European Academy of Dermatology and Venereology, the American Society for Laser Medicine and Surgery, the International Society of Dermatology, the International Hyperhidrosis Society, and the Iranian Society of Dermatology.

# Contents

# Preface

*Dermatology – The Latest Research on Common Skin Diseases* provides a comprehensive, scholarly review of common skin diseases through the lens of recent scientific advances. This volume discusses important insights into the pathophysiology, clinical outcomes, and therapeutic approaches in common skin diseases. The book includes six chapters on atopic dermatitis, vitiligo, alopecia areata, systemic scleroderma, and hidradenitis suppurativa—disorders that, despite their commonality, continue to pose significant diagnostic and therapeutic challenges.

Chapter 1, **Quality of Life Assessment in Children with Atopic Dermatitis**

This chapter comprehensively explores the multifaceted effects of Atopic Dermatitis on children's QoL, examining the physical, psychological, emotional, and social challenges faced by affected children. This review further evaluates current management strategies, including topical, systemic, and non-pharmacologic treatments, and their respective impacts on improving QoL. Despite advancements in treatment, barriers such as access to care, treatment adherence, and the chronic nature of AD continue to challenge effective QoL improvement. Future directions emphasize the importance of a multidisciplinary, patient-centered approach that incorporates emerging therapies, digital health technologies, and comprehensive psychosocial support to enhance long-term outcomes for pediatric patients with AD.

Chapter 2, **Vitiligo: Etiology and Pathophysiology**

This chapter investigates the unclear etiology of vitiligo. It is considered an autoimmune-related disease, in which autoantigens recognized by T cells from vitiligo patients were identified over the last few decades. Autoimmune reactions against melanocytes and the transfer of specific antigens are required for the development of the disease. Additionally, environmental factors may contribute to the triggering or exacerbation of lesions. Recently, oxidative stress has been identified as a modification in the micro-environment, and several stress factors can promote or inhibit the development of the disease. In terms of treatments, since several conventional treatment techniques have been established, vitiligo therapy has advanced significantly during the last few years.

Nevertheless, there is currently no permanent treatment for vitiligo. It necessitates determining which signaling pathways and target molecules are particularly compromised in vitiligo. This chapter aims to explore the etiology and pathophysiology of vitiligo and examines recent developments in vitiligo treatment, including biologics and Janus kinase (JAK) inhibitors.

Chapter 3, **Trichoscopy in the Diagnosis of Alopecia Areata**

Dermoscopy of the hair and scalp is known as trichoscopy. It is a useful method for diagnosing and monitoring hair and scalp disorders, as well as monitoring the effect of the applied treatment. The presence of exclamation mark hairs, black dots, triangular hairs, broken hairs, and pointed hairs in the alopecic patches indicates disease activity. One of the most common trichoscopic features of AA are the yellow dots - empty follicular openings filled with keratin and sebum. They predominate in long-standing, inactive diseases. Short vellus hairs are also common. The hair regrowth phase includes upright regrowing hairs and circular hairs. Diagnosis should be based on the coexistence of several trichoscopic findings rather than the presence of a single sign.

## Chapter 4, **Systemic Scleroderma: Orofacial Manifestations and Therapeutic Approaches**

This chapter examines systemic scleroderma, a multifaceted autoimmune disease that frequently presents with significant orofacial manifestations, posing substantial challenges in clinical management. Moreover, it provides a comprehensive review of the various orofacial complications associated with systemic scleroderma, including microstomia, xerostomia, periodontal disease, and temporomandibular joint disorders. The pathophysiological mechanisms underlying these manifestations are explored, highlighting the importance of early recognition and intervention. Additionally, this chapter discusses current therapeutic approaches, emphasizing the need for a multidisciplinary strategy that encompasses physical therapy, surgical options, and prosthetic rehabilitation.

## Chapter 5, **Hidradenitis Suppurativa**

This chapter provides an overview of Hidradenitis Suppurativa, including diagnostic approaches and management strategies, with a particular focus on surgical interventions. Wide local excision remains the gold standard for achieving long-term remission; however, tissue-sparing techniques, such as deroofing, offer effective alternatives, particularly in cases where post-procedural complications or cosmetic concerns are paramount. The role of advanced imaging modalities, such as ultrasound, is also discussed, emphasizing their utility in accurately assessing disease extent and guiding surgical decisions. Through a detailed case study, the importance of ultrasound guidance in identifying hidden disease processes that may elude conventional clinical evaluation is highlighted. This chapter aims to provide clinicians with a comprehensive understanding of HS, promoting informed decision-making and improved patient outcomes.

## Chapter 6, **Surgical Management of Hidradenitis Suppurativa**

This chapter focuses on surgery as an integral component of Hidradenitis Suppurativa treatment and provides an overview of different surgical techniques. Furthermore, recommendations for the surgical approach to HS patients and perioperative management are also discussed.

**Shahin Aghaei, MD**
Department of Dermatology,
School of Medicine,
Iran University of Medical Sciences,
Tehran, Iran

# Section 1

# Atopic Dermatitis

# Chapter 1

# Quality of Life Assessment in Children with Atopic Dermatitis

*Shahin Aghaei, Taha Ashouritalouki and Asma Damizadeh*

## Abstract

Atopic dermatitis (AD) is a durable inflammatory skin disorder that meaningfully influences the quality-of-life (QoL) indexes of children and the families. This review comprehensively explores the multifaceted effects of AD on QoL, examining the physical, psychological, emotional, and social challenges faced by affected children. The physical symptoms, particularly chronic pruritus and sleep disturbances, disrupt daily activities and academic performance, leading to long-term consequences on physical and cognitive development. The psychological burden of AD is profound, with children experiencing increased risks of anxiety, depression, and social isolation due to the visibility of their condition and associated stigmatization. Family dynamics are also deeply affected, as caregivers must manage the complex and ongoing demands of treatment, often resulting in significant emotional and financial stress. This review further evaluates current management strategies, including topical, systemic, and non-pharmacologic treatments, and their respective impacts on improving QoL. Despite advancements in treatment, barriers such as access to care, treatment adherence, and the chronic nature of AD continue to challenge effective QoL improvement. Future directions emphasize the importance of a multidisciplinary, patient-centered approach, incorporating emerging therapies, digital health technologies, and comprehensive psychosocial support to enhance long-term outcomes for pediatric patients with AD. This review highlights the ongoing need for innovative research and holistic management strategies to address the complex needs of this vulnerable population.

**Keywords:** quality of life, QoL, atopic dermatitis, atopic eczema, children, QoL assessment

## 1. Introduction

AD is one of the most widespread lingering inflammatory skin illnesses that affect children, with global prevalence rates ranging from 15 to 25% in pediatric populations. AD is considered by persistent itching, dry skin (xerosis), and dermatitis lesions, which can vary in severity from mild to severe. These symptoms often lead to significant physical discomfort, sleep disturbances, and an increased risk of skin infections. However, the impact of AD extends far beyond the physical manifestations of the disease. The chronic and relapsing nature of AD overwhelmingly affects the quality-of-life indexes of both the patients and their families [1, 2].

IntechOpen

In pediatric patients, QoL encompasses a broad range of factors, including physical well-being, emotional health, social interactions, and the ability to participate in normal childhood activities. The impact of AD on these aspects can be profound, leading to long-term consequences for the children's growth, education, and psychological welfare. Furthermore, the burden of managing AD also falls heavily on caregivers, who must navigate the complexities of treatment, manage flare-ups, and handle with the emotional stress connected the illness [3, 4].

This review proposes to supply an inclusive analysis of the QoL in pediatric patients with AD, examining the multifaceted impact of the disease, the effectiveness of current and emerging treatment strategies, and the challenges faced by patients and their families. By exploring the latest research and clinical trials, this review will also highlight future directions for improving the QoL of children with AD and discuss the potential of innovative therapies and multidisciplinary approaches in achieving better outcomes.

## 2. The effect of atopic dermatitis on quality-of-life index

### 2.1 Physical symptoms and their effects

One of the most challenging aspects of managing AD in children is dealing with the physical symptoms that significantly disrupt their daily lives. Chronic pruritus, or itching, is a hallmark of AD and is often the most distressing symptom for both patients and their caregivers. The constant urge to scratch can lead to skin damage, including excoriations, lichenification (thickening of the skin), and an increased risk of secondary bacterial infections, such as impetigo. These complications can exacerbate the physical discomfort associated with AD and contribute to a vicious cycle of itching and scratching [4].

Sleep disturbances are another common consequence of chronic pruritus in children with AD. Nocturnal itching often leads to frequent awakenings and poor sleep quality, which in turn results in daytime fatigue, irritability, and difficulties with concentration. These sleep disturbances can have a cascading effect on a child's daily functioning, impacting their academic performance, social interactions, and overall well-being. Studies have shown that children with AD are more likely to experience difficulties in school, have lower academic achievement, and miss more school days compared to their peers without AD [5].

In addition to sleep disturbances, the physical symptoms of AD can also affect a child's physical development and participation in physical activities. The presence of visible skin lesions may cause children to feel self-conscious or embarrassed, leading them to avoid activities that involve physical contact or exposure of their skin. This can result in reduced participation in sports, outdoor play, and other physical activities that are essential for healthy development. Moreover, the physical discomfort associated with AD may limit a child's ability to engage in regular exercise, further impacting their physical health and QoL [4].

### 2.2 Psychological and emotional impact

The psychological and emotional impact of AD on pediatric patients is profound. Children patients with AD are at an amplified risk of emerging anxiety, depression, and other psychological disorders due to the chronic nature of the disease and the associated physical discomfort. The visible symptoms of AD, such as inflamed and scaly skin, can lead to feelings of embarrassment, low self-esteem, and social withdrawal. This emotional burden is often compounded by the stigmatization that children with AD may face, particularly in social settings such as school, where appearance can play a significant role in peer acceptance [3, 4].

Adolescents with AD are particularly vulnerable to the psychological effects of the disease. During this critical period of social development, the pressure to conform to social norms and maintain a positive self-image is intense. The presence of visible skin lesions can make adolescents feel self-conscious, leading to social isolation and a decreased sense of belonging. This can have long-term implications for their mental health and overall QoL [3, 4].

In younger children, the emotional impact of AD may manifest differently, with increased irritability, temper tantrums, and difficulties in managing emotions. These behavioral challenges can strain relationships with caregivers and peers, leading to further social isolation and emotional distress. The chronic nature of AD means that these psychological and emotional challenges are not limited to periods of flare-ups but may persist even during periods of remission, as the fear of recurrence and the burden of ongoing treatment weigh heavily on the child [3, 4].

## 2.3 Social and behavioral effects

AD also has substantial social and behavioral implications for pediatric patients. The need for regular treatment, including the application of topical medications and frequent visits to healthcare providers, can interfere with school attendance and participation in extracurricular activities. The chronic nature of the disease can lead to missed school days, reduced academic performance, and difficulties in maintaining consistent participation in social activities [3, 4].

Behavioral issues such as irritability, temper tantrums, and difficulty managing emotions are not uncommon in children with chronic AD. These behaviors may stem from the constant discomfort and frustration associated with the disease, as well as the challenges of adhering to a demanding treatment regimen. Such behavioral challenges can strain relationships with peers, teachers, and family members, further impacting the child's social life and overall QoL [4, 6].

The impact of AD on social development can be particularly pronounced during adolescence, a time when peer relationships and social acceptance are crucial. Adolescents with AD may experience bullying or teasing due to their appearance, leading to further social withdrawal and isolation. This can have a lasting impact on their self-esteem and social skills, potentially affecting their ability to form and maintain relationships in adulthood [3, 4].

## 2.4 Family dynamics and caregiver burden

The burden of AD extends beyond the affected child to their family members, particularly caregivers. Managing a child's AD often requires significant time, effort, and financial resources. Caregivers are responsible for administering treatments, managing flare-ups, and attending frequent medical appointments, all of which can lead to physical and emotional exhaustion. The chronic nature of AD means that these caregiving demands are ongoing, leading to sustained stress that can affect family dynamics and the overall QoL of the family [4, 7].

Financial strain is another significant burden for families managing pediatric AD. The cost of medications, special skincare products, and other necessary treatments can add up, particularly if the child's condition is severe and requires more intensive management. Additionally, caregivers may experience lost productivity or income due to the need to care for their child, further exacerbating the financial impact of the disease [7].

Parents and caregivers often experience feelings of guilt, anxiety, and helplessness, particularly when conventional treatments fail to provide relief for their child. These emotional burdens can lead to caregiver burnout, which in turn can negatively affect the entire family's dynamics and QoL. The stress associated with managing a chronic, relapsing condition like AD can take a toll on the mental health of both the child and their caregivers, making comprehensive support essential for improving QoL [7].

The impact of AD on family dynamics can also extend to siblings, who may feel neglected or resentful due to the attention focused on the affected child. Siblings may also experience anxiety or distress related to the unpredictability of the disease and the emotional strain it places on the family. Addressing the needs of the entire family, including providing support for siblings, is an important aspect of managing pediatric AD and improving overall QoL [7].

## 3. Assessing quality of life in pediatric atopic dermatitis

### 3.1 QoL measurement tools and their application

Assessing QoL in pediatric patients with AD is critical for understanding the full impact of the disease and tailoring treatment plans accordingly. Several tools have been developed to measure QoL in children with skin conditions, each offering unique insights into the patient's experience.

The Children's Dermatology Life Quality Index (CDLQI) is one of the most commonly utilized instruments for assessing QoL in pediatric patients with dermatological conditions, including AD. The CDLQI measures the effect of the illness on various parts of life, including symptoms, daily activities, school performance, and social interactions. This tool provides valuable information on how the disease affects the child's life from their perspective, helping healthcare providers tailor interventions to improve QoL [3].

The Dermatology Life Quality Index (DLQI) is another widely used tool, although it is more commonly applied to adult populations. The DLQI assesses similar domains as the CDLQI but is tailored to older patients, making it less suitable for younger children. However, it remains a valuable tool for assessing the impact of AD on older adolescents, who may experience different challenges compared to younger children [3].

The Patient-Oriented Eczema Measure (POEM) and the Scoring Atopic Dermatitis (SCORAD) index are also valuable tools for assessing disease severity and its correlation with QoL. POEM is a patient-reported outcome measure that captures the frequency of key symptoms, such as itching and sleep disturbance, while SCORAD combines both clinical assessment and patient-reported symptoms to provide a comprehensive view of disease severity. These tools are particularly useful for monitoring the effectiveness of treatment and making adjustments to improve QoL [3, 5, 6].

### 3.2 Challenges in QoL assessment across age groups

Assessing QoL in pediatric patients presents unique challenges, particularly when dealing with diverse age sets. Junior children might not fully understand or articulate how their condition affects them, requiring caregivers to provide proxy responses. While proxy reports are valuable, they may not fully capture the child's subjective experience, leading to potential discrepancies between caregiver and patient perceptions of QoL [4, 5].

Adolescents, on the other hand, may have a better understanding of their condition and its impact on their lives. However, they may also experience heightened emotional distress due to the social implications of visible skin lesions. Adolescence is a critical period for social development, and the stigmatization associated with AD can have a profound impact on self-esteem and social relationships. Therefore, it is essential to use age-appropriate QoL assessment tools that consider the unique challenges faced by different age groups [4, 5].

Understanding the developmental stages of children is also important in QoL assessment. For example, younger children may be more focused on the physical discomfort associated with AD, while older children and adolescents may be more concerned with the social and emotional aspects of the disease. Tailoring QoL assessments to these developmental stages can provide a more accurate picture of how AD impacts the child's life and help guide treatment decisions [4, 5].

## 4. Current management strategies for pediatric AD and their impact on QoL

### 4.1 Topical treatments: Effectiveness and QoL outcomes

Topical corticosteroids (TCS) and topical calcineurin inhibitors (TCIs) are the backbone of AD treatment, particularly for managing acute flares and maintaining disease control. These treatments are effective in reducing inflammation and pruritus, leading to significant improvements in QoL. However, concerns about the side effects of long-term TCS use, such as skin thinning and adrenal suppression, can lead to "steroid phobia," resulting in underuse and suboptimal disease control [8–10].

TCIs, such as tacrolimus and pimecrolimus, offer a steroid-sparing alternative, particularly for sensitive areas like the face and neck. They have been shown to improve QoL by effectively managing symptoms without the risk of skin atrophy. However, their use is often limited by concerns about long-term safety, particularly the theoretical risk of malignancy, which has not been substantiated by robust clinical evidence [9].

The regular use of moisturizers and emollients is also critical for maintaining skin barrier function, preventing flare-ups, and reducing the frequency of TCS use. These non-pharmacologic interventions are particularly important for long-term disease management and can significantly improve QoL by reducing the physical discomfort associated with dry, itchy skin [11].

The impact of these treatments on QoL is closely tied to patient adherence. Ensuring that families understand the importance of regular application and are comfortable with the use of topical treatments is essential for achieving optimal outcomes. Addressing concerns about side effects and providing clear guidance on the safe use of these treatments can help improve adherence and, consequently, QoL [6].

### 4.2 Systemic treatments and QoL improvements

For children with severe, treatment-resistant AD, systemic therapies such as omalizumab, biologics, and JAK inhibitors offer new hope. Omalizumab, an anti-IgE monoclonal antibody, has been shown in clinical trials to significantly reduce the severity of AD and improve QoL by reducing the need for potent TCS and improving overall disease management. This treatment is particularly beneficial for patients with high IgE levels who have not responded to conventional therapies [12].

Biologics, such as dupilumab, which targets specific cytokines involved in the inflammatory process, have also demonstrated significant improvements in both disease severity and QoL. These therapies provide a targeted approach to treatment, reducing the systemic side effects associated with traditional immunosuppressants. However, they are not without risks, and their impact on QoL must be balanced against potential adverse effects, including injection site reactions and the need for ongoing monitoring [13, 14].

JAK inhibitors, another class of systemic therapies, offer promise in managing severe AD by targeting key signaling pathways involved in inflammation. These treatments have shown efficacy in reducing symptoms and improving QoL in clinical trials, although their long-term safety and effectiveness in pediatric populations remain areas of active research [1, 2].

The impact of systemic treatments on QoL is particularly significant for children with severe AD, who may experience profound improvements in their physical symptoms, emotional well-being, and social interactions as a result of these therapies. However, the high cost of biologics and other systemic treatments can be a barrier to access, particularly for families without adequate insurance coverage. Ensuring that all children have access to these potentially life-changing therapies is a critical challenge in improving QoL for pediatric AD patients [15].

### 4.3 Non-pharmacologic interventions

Non-pharmacologic interventions play a crucial role in managing AD and improving QoL. Regular use of moisturizers and emollients is essential for maintaining skin barrier function, preventing flare-ups, and reducing the frequency of TCS use. These interventions are particularly important for long-term disease management and can significantly improve QoL by reducing the physical discomfort associated with dry, itchy skin [11].

Dietary modifications and environmental control measures, such as avoiding known allergens and irritants, can also help manage AD and improve QoL. While the evidence supporting these interventions is mixed, they may be beneficial for some patients, particularly those with known food allergies or sensitivities. Identifying and eliminating potential triggers from the child's environment can reduce the frequency and severity of flare-ups, leading to better disease control and improved QoL [16].

Psychosocial support and educational interventions are critical components of comprehensive AD management. Educating patients and their families about the nature of the disease, treatment options, and proper skin care techniques empowers them to take control of the condition and improves adherence to treatment plans. Psychosocial care, together with counseling and groups' care, can help families deal with the sensitive and communal encounters associated with AD, leading to better overall QoL outcomes [3].

In addition to traditional interventions, complementary and alternative medicine approaches, such as acupuncture, herbal remedies, and relaxation techniques, are increasingly being explored as adjuncts to conventional treatments. While the evidence supporting these approaches is still limited, some families find them helpful in managing symptoms and improving QoL. Integrating these approaches into a holistic treatment plan, when appropriate, can provide additional options for families seeking to improve their child's QoL [16].

## 4.4 Real-world applications and case studies

The Atopic Dermatitis Anti-IgE Pediatric Trial (ADAPT) provides a compelling case study on the usage of omalizumab in children with a severe form of disease, treatment-resistant AD. The trial demonstrated that omalizumab significantly reduced disease severity and improved QoL, particularly in children with high IgE levels who had not responded to other treatments. The corticosteroid-sparing effect observed in the trial suggests that omalizumab could reduce the long-term side effects associated with TCS use, further enhancing QoL [12].

In this study, participants who received omalizumab reported significant improvements in QoL, including reduced itching, better sleep quality, and less emotional distress. These improvements were accompanied by a decrease in the use of potent TCS, indicating that omalizumab not only provided symptom relief but also helped maintain disease control with a lower treatment burden. The positive outcomes observed in the ADAPT trial underscore the efficacy of omalizumab as a valuable therapy option for severe pediatric AD, particularly in cases where conventional therapies have failed [12].

The efficacy of dupilumab, another biologic, in improving QoL in pediatric AD patients has also been demonstrated in clinical trials. Dupilumab has been shown to significantly reduce the severity of AD, improve sleep quality, and enhance overall well-being, making it a promising option for children with moderate to severe forms of AD. These findings highlight the potential of biologics to transform the management of pediatric AD and improve the lives of affected children [13, 14].

In real-world settings, the impact of these therapies on QoL can vary depending on factors such as access to care, adherence to treatment, and the presence of comorbid conditions. Case studies and observational studies can provide valuable insights into how these therapies perform outside of controlled clinical trials, helping to inform treatment decisions and improve patient outcomes.

## 5. Challenges in improving quality of life in pediatric AD

### 5.1 Access to care: Barriers and disparities

Regardless of the accessibility of efficacious treatments, numerous children with AD face barriers to accessing care, particularly those from low-income families or underserved communities. Disparities in access to emerging therapies, such as biologics and JAK inhibitors, can exacerbate health inequities and result in suboptimal QoL outcomes for some patients. Financial barriers, including the high cost of medications and limited insurance coverage, can also limit access to care, leading to gaps in treatment and disease management [1, 4].

The high cost of emerging therapies, such as biologics, poses a significant challenge for many families. While these treatments offer significant improvements in QoL, their affordability remains a concern. Insurance coverage for these therapies varies, and out-of-pocket costs can be prohibitively high for some families. This financial burden can prevent children from receiving the most effective treatments, leading to poorer QoL outcomes and increased disease burden [1, 7].

Geographic disparities also play a role in admittance to repair. Patient children residing in country areas may have partial access to dermatologists and other specialists, making it more difficult to receive timely and appropriate care. Telemedicine has the potential to address some of these challenges by providing remote access to specialist care, but barriers such as limited Internet access and technological literacy can still impede the use of these services in underserved communities [1].

## 5.2 Adherence to treatment: Enhancing outcomes

Treatment adherence is a critical factor in achieving optimal outcomes in pediatric AD. However, adherence can be challenging, particularly in young children who may resist frequent application of topical treatments or in families who struggle to maintain consistent treatment routines. Factors affecting adherence include the complexity of the treatment regimen, the burden of daily care, and concerns about side effects. Strategies to improve adherence, such as simplifying treatment regimens, providing clear instructions, and offering psychosocial support, are essential for enhancing QoL in pediatric patients [3, 6].

For example, simplifying treatment regimens by using combination therapies or long-acting medications can reduce the treatment burden on families and improve adherence. Providing clear, age-appropriate instructions and educational materials can also help children and their caregivers better understand the importance of adherence and how to manage their condition effectively. Psychosocial support, including counseling and support groups, can help families cope with the challenges of managing a chronic condition like AD and improve adherence to treatment plans [3, 6].

## 5.3 Long-term disease management, monitoring, and the burden of chronicity

Managing AD as a chronic condition requires ongoing monitoring and adjustment of treatment plans to address changes in disease severity and patient needs. Long-term management is particularly challenging in pediatric populations, as the disease may evolve, necessitating changes in treatment strategy. Regular follow-up visits, comprehensive care plans, and patient-centered approaches are critical for ensuring that QoL remains a priority throughout the disease [11].

Long-term management also involves addressing comorbidities and preventing relapse. Children with AD are at augmented risk for evolving other atopic conditions, such as asthma and allergic rhinitis, which can have more impact on their QoL. Managing these comorbidities effectively requires a multidisciplinary approach that includes allergists, dermatologists, pediatricians, and other specialists working together to provide comprehensive care. Preventing relapse is also a key component of long-term management, as flare-ups can lead to significant declines in QoL and increased disease burden [4, 11].

Psychological support for children and families dealing with the chronic nature of AD is also essential. The ongoing nature of the disease can lead to feelings of helplessness, frustration, and burnout, particularly when flare-ups occur despite treatment adherence. Providing ongoing psychosocial support, including counseling, stress management techniques, and support groups, can help families cope with the emotional toll of the disease and maintain a positive outlook on treatment and management [3, 11].

# 6. Future directions in enhancing QoL for pediatric AD patients

## 6.1 Innovations in treatment approaches

The landscape of AD treatment is rapidly evolving, with new therapies offering the potential to significantly improve QoL for pediatric patients. Advances in biologics and targeted therapies, such as JAK inhibitors and anti-IgE monoclonal antibodies, represent a shift toward more personalized and effective treatment options. These therapies target specific pathways involved in AD pathogenesis, providing a more focused approach to disease management with potentially fewer side effects compared to traditional systemic treatments [1].

Emerging non-pharmacologic strategies, such as the use of probiotics, microbiome-based therapies, and personalized medicine approaches, are also being explored as potential avenues for improving QoL in pediatric AD patients. These approaches aim to address the underlying causes of AD and restore balance to the immune system and skin microbiome, offering a more holistic approach to disease management. Although these therapies are still in the primary stages of investigations, they clutch capacities for giving new treatment options that are less reliant on pharmacologic interventions [16].

## 6.2 Integrating multidisciplinary care into standard practice

The importance of a multidisciplinary approach in managing pediatric AD cannot be overstated. Children with severe or complex AD often require care from a team of specialists, including dermatologists, allergists, pediatricians, psychologists, and other healthcare providers. This team-based method guarantees that all characteristics of the child's health are addressed, from managing physical symptoms to providing psychological support and addressing comorbid conditions [11].

Integrating multidisciplinary care into standard practice involves coordinating care across different specialties, ensuring that all providers are working together to achieve the best possible outcomes for the child. This approach can help prevent fragmentation of care, reduce the risk of missed diagnoses or treatment delays, and provide a more comprehensive, patient-centered approach to managing pediatric AD [11].

In addition to specialist care, primary care providers play a critical role in managing pediatric AD. They are frequently the initial point of connection for families and are in authority for coordinating care, monitoring treatment progress, and providing ongoing support. Ensuring that primary care providers have the necessary training and resources to manage pediatric AD effectively is essential for improving QoL and long-term outcomes [11].

## 6.3 Patient-centered research and future studies

Despite significant advances in AD treatment, there are still many unanswered questions regarding the long-lasing protection and efficiency of emerging therapies, particularly in pediatric populations. Additional study is needed to explore the effect of these treatments on QoL, as well as to identify potential biomarkers that can guide personalized treatment strategies. Additionally, supplementary research is needed to evaluate the effectiveness of non-pharmacologic interventions, such as dietary modifications and psychosocial support, in improving QoL for children with AD [1, 11].

The role of patient-centered research in shaping future treatment guidelines cannot be overstated. Understanding the patient and family perspectives on treatment outcomes, adherence, and QoL will be essential for developing guidelines that are both effective and feasible in real-world settings. Future research should also focus on the long-term impact of emerging therapies on different subgroups of pediatric patients, including those with varying levels of disease severity and comorbid conditions [1, 3].

Engaging patients and families in the research process, through initiatives such as patient-reported outcomes and participatory research, can help ensure that future studies are aligned with the needs and priorities of those affected by AD. This approach can lead to the development of more effective, patient-centered treatment strategies that improve QoL and long-term outcomes for pediatric AD patients [5].

## 7. Conclusion

The quality-of-life index in children with atopic dermatitis is deeply influenced by emotional, physical and social encounters related to this disease. While traditional therapies remain the cornerstone of AD management, emerging therapies offer new hope for improving quality of life, particularly in children with severe or refractory disease. A comprehensive and patient-centered approach that includes pharmacological and non-pharmacological interventions, psychosocial support, and patient education is necessary to achieve long-term disease control and increase quality of life indicators for children with atopic eczema. As research continues to progress, the future holds promise for further improvements in the management and quality of life of pediatric AD patients.

## Acknowledgements

The authors acknowledge the usage of ChatGPT-4o for language polishing of the manuscript.

## Author details

Shahin Aghaei*, Taha Ashouritalouki and Asma Damizadeh
Department of Dermatology, School of Medicine, Iran University of Medical Sciences, Tehran, Iran

*Address all correspondence to: shahinaghaei@yahoo.com

## IntechOpen

# References

[1] Johnson H, Yu J. Current and emerging therapies in pediatric atopic dermatitis. Dermatology and Therapy (Heidelb). 2022;**12**(12):2691-2703

[2] Kondratuk K, Netravali IA, Castelo-Soccio L. Modern interventions for pediatric atopic dermatitis: An updated pharmacologic approach. Dermatology and Therapy (Heidelb). 2023;**13**:367-389

[3] Zhao M, Liang Y, Shen C, Wang Y, Ma L, Ma X. Patient education programs in pediatric atopic dermatitis: A systematic review of randomized controlled trials and meta-analysis. Dermatology and Therapy (Heidelb). 2020;**10**(3):449-464

[4] Kisieliene I, Mainelis A, Rudzeviciene O, Bylaite-Bucinskiene M, Wollenberg A. The burden of pediatric atopic dermatitis: Quality of life of patients and their families. Journal of Clinical Medicine. 2024;**13**(6):1700

[5] Fishbein AB, Lora J, Penedo FJ, Forrest CB, Griffith JW, Paller AS. Patient-reported outcomes for measuring sleep disturbance in pediatric atopic dermatitis: Cross-sectional study of PROMIS pediatric sleep measures and actigraphy. Journal of the American Academy of Dermatology. 2023;**88**(2):348-356

[6] Bass AM, Anderson KL, Feldman SR. Interventions to increase treatment adherence in pediatric atopic dermatitis: A systematic review. Journal of Clinical Medicine. 2015;**4**(2):231-242

[7] Saeki H, Ohya Y, Nawata H, Arima K, Inukai M, Rossi AB, et al. Impact of the family and household environment on pediatric atopic dermatitis in Japan. Journal of Clinical Medicine. 2023;**12**(8):2988

[8] Andre N, Ben Shmuel A, Yahav L, Muallem L, Golan Tripto I, Horev A. Is corticophobia spreading among pediatricians? Insights from a self-efficacy survey on the management of pediatric atopic dermatitis. Translational Pediatrics. 2023;**12**(10):1823-1834

[9] Ohtsuki M, Morimoto H, Nakagawa H. Tacrolimus ointment for the treatment of adult and pediatric atopic dermatitis: Review on safety and benefits. The Journal of Dermatology. 2018;**45**(8):936-942

[10] Kamiya K, Saeki H, Tokura Y, Yoshihara S, Sugai J, Ohtsuki M. Proactive versus rank-down topical corticosteroid therapy for maintenance of remission in pediatric atopic dermatitis: A randomized, open-label, active-controlled, parallel-group study (anticipate study). Journal of Clinical Medicine. 2022;**11**(21):6477

[11] Naik PP. Recent insights into the management of treatment-resistant pediatric atopic dermatitis. International Journal of Women's Dermatology. 2022;**8**:e023

[12] Chan S, Cornelius V, Cro S, Harper JI, Lack G. Treatment effect of omalizumab on severe pediatric atopic dermatitis: The ADAPT randomized clinical trial. JAMA Pediatrics. 2020;**174**(1):29-37

[13] Kamphuis E, Boesjes CM, Loman L, Bakker DS, Poelhekken M, Zuithoff NPA, et al. Dupilumab in daily practice for the treatment of pediatric atopic dermatitis: 28-week clinical and biomarker results from the

BioDay registry. Pediatric Allergy and Immunology. 2022;**33**:e13887

[14] Belmesk L, Hatami A, Powell J, Kokta V, Coulombe J. Successful use of dupilumab in recalcitrant pediatric atopic dermatitis-like graft-versus-host disease: A case series. JAAD Case Reports. 2024;**44**:11-16

[15] Zhao A, Pan C, Li M. Biologics and oral small-molecule inhibitors for treatment of pediatric atopic dermatitis: Opportunities and challenges. Pediatric Investigation. 2023;**7**(3):177-190

[16] Dimitriades VR, Wisner E. Treating pediatric atopic dermatitis: Current perspectives. Pediatric Health, Medicine and Therapeutics. 2015;**6**:93-99

# Section 2

# Vitiligo

Chapter 2

# Vitiligo: Etiology and Pathophysiology

*Rawan Almutairi*

## Abstract

Vitiligo's etiology is still unclear and remains the subject of many studies. It is considered to be an autoimmune-related disease in which autoantigens recognized by T cells from the vitiligo patient were identified during the last decades. Autoimmune reactions against melanocytes and the transfer of specific antigens are required for the development of the disease. In addition, environmental factors may be involved in vitiligo's triggering or facilitating the appearance of lesions. Recently, oxidative stress has been identified as a modification in the microenvironment, and several stress factors can promote or inhibit the development of the disease. In terms of treatments, since a number of conventional treatment techniques have been established, vitiligo therapy has advanced significantly during the last few years. Nevertheless, there is currently no permanent treatment for vitiligo. It necessitates determining which signaling pathways and target molecules are particularly compromised in vitiligo. This chapter intends to address the etiology and pathophysiology of vitiligo, and attempts to address new developments in vitiligo treatment, particularly biologics and Janus kinases (JAK) inhibitors.

**Keywords:** vitiligo, pigmentation, autoimmunity, oxidative stress, leukoderma

## 1. Introduction

The exact etiology of vitiligo is not known. It is considered to be a multifactorial polygenic disorder, which develops when genetically predisposed individuals are exposed to accelerating factors like stress and infections. From the time when the first reports of this disease were made, different theories of the mechanism of vitiligo in the human body have been established. Despite the long observation period and plenty of reported data, there is no single theory that can elucidate the mystery of vitiligo pathomechanism. There have been many explanations of the causes of vitiligo, most of which cannot completely elucidate the mystery of this complex immunologically mediated disorder. With a great increase in basic and clinical immunological research, growing evidence suggests that skin depigmentation in the affected areas is caused by autoimmunity to melanocytes [1, 2].

In the past decade, the management of vitiligo has shown great progress with the establishment of several standard treatment modalities. However, the long-term cure for vitiligo is still lacking. It requires identifying the target molecules and the signaling pathways that are primarily defective in vitiligo. This chapter intends to address the etiology and pathophysiology of vitiligo, overviewing important topics like genetic factors, the autoimmunity in vitiligo, the role of melanocytes, the immune privilege of melanocytes, and the trigger of oxidative stress and each of these environments in the pathophysiology of vitiligo. This chapter also aims to discuss the emerging therapy in the field of vitiligo, specifically JAK inhibitors and Biologics.

## 2. Genetic factors in vitiligo

The significance of genetic factors in the development of vitiligo is strongly supported by an extensive number of studies, despite the fact that these influences are complicated. Vitiligo's tendency to develop within families has been demonstrated by extensive epidemiological investigations; nevertheless, the genetic susceptibility is not absolute [3–5]. The vast majority of vitiligo cases (91%) do not have known close relatives afflicted by vitiligo, while 9% of vitiligo cases have multiple close relatives with vitiligo (multiplex). The heritability of vitiligo, which relates to the proportion of the total vitiligo risk that is due to genetic variation, is exceedingly high. In fact, genetic factors are responsible for approximately 80% of the vitiligo risk, while the remaining 20% is attributed to environmental factors [6]. A number of loci and candidate genes have been identified as a consequence of genome-wide linkage analyses conducted in multiple patient populations. Numerous of these genes are responsible for melanogenesis, immune regulation, or apoptosis and have been linked to other pigmentary, autoinflammatory, or autoimmune disorders [7–9].

## 3. Pathophysiology of vitiligo

### 3.1 Melanocyte dysfunction

The etiology and pathogenesis of vitiligo result from complex genetics, biochemical pathways, and cellular mechanisms. Although a clear understanding remains elusive, the dysregulation of both immune and biochemical pathways that are crucial for maintaining melanocyte cellular homeostasis and survival is essential. These mechanisms include genetic/epigenetic components, oxidative stress, altered proinflammatory cytokines, and soluble factors that may trigger the disease. Melanocyte autoimmune behaviors are targets that can trigger the destruction of melanocyte epitopes through loss of cellular immune tolerance resulting in an immune response [10]. This apoptotic deterioration is facilitated by a combination of poor antioxidant defense and elevated reactive oxygen species levels. The genes that have been well-studied in this context are those encoding the melanocyte antigen, premelanosome protein, melanosomal proteins that serve as autoantigens, and proteins governing oxidative stress control. Taken together, the resulting sequence of pathogenic melanocyte dysfunction is orchestrated by a combination of heightened melanogenic activity and melanocyte-specific oxidative stress, inefficient melanin synthesis and accumulation, ineffective cessation of autoimmune reactions, and ultimate melanocyte cell death [11, 12].

### 3.2 Cellular and molecular mechanisms

The loss of functioning melanocytes leading to vitiligo development has been considered to be an autoimmune process. This has been supported by several major clinical and experimental clues. One of the earliest indications supporting the auto-immune hypothesis in vitiligo was the perivascular lymphocytic infiltration at the lesional sites. The histology of active vitiligo demonstrated an increase of activated cytotoxic T cells and macrophages, indicating the recruitment of effector lympho-cytes to the skin. The relationship between vitiligo onset and episodic stress, as well as the correlation between autoimmune diseases and vitiligo, has indicated the partici-pation of autoimmune responses in the progression of the disease [13].

The hypothesis of autoimmune participation in vitiligo is further supported by the convincing evidence of innate and adaptive immunity enhancement at both the lesional sites in active and stable vitiligo, and even in normal-appearing skin from vitiliginous patients [14]. The data from the human skin microarray analysis have substantiated that for lesional skin, classic Th1-differentiation chemokines like CXCL9/10/11 play the most important impacts. For non-lesional skin, the microarray data have suggested the role of melanocyte apoptosis in continuous immune response induction by enriching genes that are expressed during apoptotic processes, but not through facilitating chemotaxis- or immune reactive cell regulators. There are many molecules that could induce melanocyte death in the borderline of intact and depig-menting skin, including tumor necrosis factor-alpha (TNF-$\alpha$) and histamine [13–16].

### 3.3 Oxidative stress

The most widely accepted theory for the progressive skin hypopigmentation observed in patients with vitiligo is the oxidative stress theory, which supposes that reactive oxygen species may cause melanocyte dysfunction, resulting in the loss of melanocytes and consequent skin depigmentation. Generation of toxic levels of superoxide radicals and hydrogen peroxide, inhibitors and/or decreases of produc-tions of tyrosine and tyrosinase, a glycosylated active-site form of the copper-con-taining enzyme tyrosinase, increased sensitivity of melanocytes to $H_2O_2$, abnormal premature aging of melanocytes, a loss of balance between the generation of free radicals and scavenging antioxidant defenses, and defective repair system for oxida-tively damaged melanocytes all have been postulated for vitiligo pathogenesis [17–19].

### 3.4 Cytokine imbalance

Cytokines are soluble protein molecules that control cell growth and differentia-tion. They are classified based on their relationship to the immune system as well as their function and structure. Molecules that stimulate the immune system are termed cytokines, and those that inhibit immune processes are called cytokine antagonists. In most instances, cytokines are mostly polypeptides produced locally near their site of action and do not represent a highly selective and potent targeting compound. Hence, one cytokine can affect various target cells, depending on the receptors expressed by these cells, delivering multiple signals, and consequently, cytokines can also have multiple biological functions. On the other hand, the effects of stimulation by different cytokines are regulated by the stages of cellular differ-entiation and the relative expression of various cytokine receptors [20]. Therefore, additional studies on cytokines and cytokine receptor families are being carried out to understand the relevant signaling pathways. To date, over 80 cytokines have been reported. Among the large array of cytokines, it seems that only a few play signifi-cant roles in the pathogenesis of several autoimmune diseases, such as IL-6, IL-12, IL-18, TNF-$\alpha$, IL-10, and IFN-$\gamma$ [21].

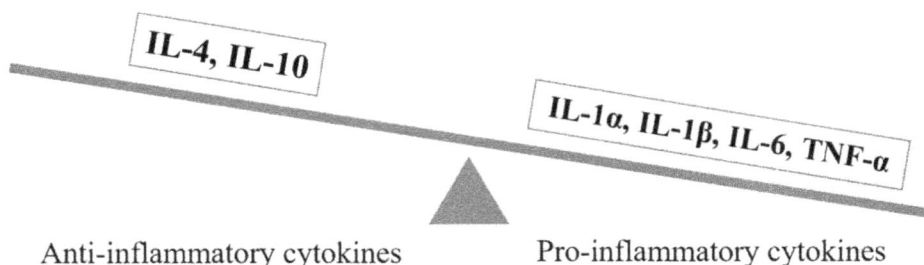

**IL-4, IL-10**

**IL-1α, IL-1β, IL-6, TNF-α**

Anti-inflammatory cytokines      Pro-inflammatory cytokines

**Figure 1.**
*Cytokine imbalance enhances the susceptibility of melanocyte destruction in vitiligo. TNF, Tumor necrosis factor; IL, interleukin.*

Several studies have demonstrated proinflammatory cytokines, such as IL-1α, IL-1β, and TNF-α, to act as critical determinants of cell-mediated immunity and to be involved in the regulation of skin pigmentation **Figure 1**, [22]. Many of these cytokines are elevated in the sera of vitiligo patients and, importantly, in lesional tissue. The underlying inflammatory response appears to lead to the overproduction of reactive oxygen species and serum nitric oxide levels in many patients. Conversely, other cytokines, including IL-10, which has an inhibitory effect on cell-mediated immunity, have been shown to be reduced in both patients' sera and lesional areas. The depletion of regulatory T cells in the skin lesion of vitiligo may also allow for a lymphocyte reaction to ultimately lead to melanocyte cytotoxicity. The pivotal role of cytokines underlying vitiligo pathogenesis has been further illustrated in preclinical and pilot experimental therapeutic studies using monoclonal antibodies targeting the aforementioned cytokines, suggesting that the process is reversible [23].

## 4. Environmental triggers

Environmental factors have been implicated in the etiology and pathogenesis of vitiligo. Indeed, environmental factors such as exposure to sunburn damage, contact with certain chemicals, cosmetic products, or trauma at several cutaneous sites are involved in vitiligo pathogenesis. The depletion of cutaneous protective factors such as phenolic compounds, vitamins, and several cytokines could also be involved in the pathogenesis of the disease. Several reports have indicated that tyrosine metabolism is affected by ultraviolet radiation, which explains the plethora of antioxidants used in the therapy of vitiligo. Moreover, certain chemicals and cosmetics have been incriminated as suppressive agents in regulating innate and adaptive immune responses induced by ultraviolet radiation [1].

### 4.1 Chemical exposure

Chemical-associated vitiligo, also known as leukoderma, has been documented in rubber industry workers who are exposed to phenolic compounds. The initial agent to be identified was hydroquinone monobenzyl ether (monobenzone), which induces cell death without activating the caspase cascade or DNA fragmentation [24]. Rhododendrol, an additional phenolic compound that is utilized in skin-lightening treatments and was responsible for an outbreak of leukoderma in Japan, induces cytotoxicity through a tyrosinase-dependent mechanism [25]. The appearance of leukoderma has also been linked to hair pigments, with paraphenylenediamine being one of the primary suspects. Nevertheless, the causal mechanism by which benzene derivatives induce depigmentation has not yet been determined [26, 27].

## 5. Emerging treatments of vitiligo

### 5.1 Janus kinase inhibitors

Janus kinases (JAKs) are a family of tyrosine kinases operating within the Janus kinase/signal transducer and activator of the transcription (JAK/STAT) pathway, which plays an important role in immune regulation. The exact mechanism of how JAK inhibitors reduce the autoimmunity-associated destruction of melanocytes has not been fully established, but it is thought that the dominant role of these inhibitors is in suppressing the inflammatory part of this process, and not the actual repigmentation [28]. By facilitating a switch to lesional skin repigmentation, the repigmentation can be completed using a variety of repigmentation strategies. Ruxolitinib cream 1.5% (Opzelura), a potent and selective JAK1 and JAK2 inhibitor, is a newly approved medication for use in patients aged ≥ 12 years with non-segmental vitiligo [29]. The clinical significance of these molecules as a new era of vitiligo treatment for both unique and combination treatment options is beginning to be recognized. The understanding of vitiligo has evolved greatly over the past decades, and JAK inhibitors have revolutionized the approach to this condition, even adding a component to their pathomechanism. JAK inhibitors have been successful in treating significant and generalized vitiligo, a very difficult and recalcitrant disease, primarily in adults [30].

### 5.2 Biologics

Biological treatments for vitiligo are being explored, and several types have shown promise, although the evidence is still evolving. These biological agents are some kind of monoclonal antibodies, proteins that are produced by recombinant DNA technology, directed at defined molecular targets, and may have potential in treating vitiligo. Based on the abnormal immune responses and alterations in cytokine levels observed in vitiligo patients, it is possible that targeting proinflammatory mediators, such as TNF and ILs-12, 23, and 17, could be a promising treatment strategy. TNF-α inhibitors, such as infliximab, adalimumab, and etanercept, have been tried in a few cases. However, the results are mixed and inconclusive. Some studies reported no repigmentation or even worsening of the condition, while others observed improvement in refractory cases. Ustekinumab, which targets IL-12 and IL-23, has been used in some cases. While it improved psoriasis in a patient with concomitant vitiligo, it did not consistently improve vitiligo and in some cases led to new lesions. There is limited evidence on the use of IL-17 inhibitors in vitiligo. However, given the role of IL-17 in autoimmune diseases, it is an area of ongoing research [30].

### 5.3 Gene therapy

Conventional vitiligo treatments have the potential to control the disease and repigment the depigmented skin. But often, these are unresponsive, offer a slow response, or require long-term therapy. Researchers continually search for an ideal treatment to fully recover skin pigmentation in an effective and lasting manner. In this regard, gene therapy is a novel treatment, and much research is being conducted as an initiation of gene therapies. In vitiligo, there are both localized patches and generalized skin disease conditions. Both localized and generalized vitiligo cause premature hair whitening (trichrome vitiligo). Moreover, most gene therapy studies have been conducted to treat localized patches alone but not generalized vitiligo along with hair repigmentation. Gene therapy aims to deliver a gene of interest directly to the defected skin area to ameliorate the disease condition. For the development of gene therapies, major challenges still need to be addressed, and it has remained an emerging field in vitiligo.

## 6. Conclusion

In summary, vitiligo likely results from an interaction of genetic susceptibility, autoimmunity, oxidative stress, and environmental factors that lead to melanocyte dysfunction and destruction. The exact mechanisms integrating these various pathways are still not fully elucidated. An enhanced understanding of the pathophysiology of vitiligo is key to enabling the development of new, effective, and safe treatments for a previously recalcitrant condition with a great psychoemotional impact on its sufferers. Although further research is necessary on the new emerging treatments including JAK inhibitors and biologics, these potential treatments warrant hope in improving the disease course of vitiligo.

## Appendices and nomenclature

| | |
|---|---|
| DNA | deoxyribonucleic acid |
| TNF-α | tumor necrosis factor-alpha |
| IL | interleukin |
| JAK | Janus kinase |
| STAT | signal transducer and activator of transcription |

## Author details

Rawan Almutairi
Dermatology Department, Farwaniya Hospital, Farwaniya Government, Kuwait

*Address all correspondence to: r.mutairi95@hotmail.com

## IntechOpen

# References

[1] Bergqvist C, Ezzedine K. Vitiligo: A review. Dermatology. 2020;**236**(6):571-592. DOI: 10.1159/000506103

[2] Frisoli ML, Essien K, Harris JE. Vitiligo: Mechanisms of pathogenesis and treatment. Annual Review of Immunology. 2020;**38**:621-648. DOI: 10.1146/annurev-immunol-100919-023531

[3] Majumder PP, Nordlund JJ, Nath SK. Pattern of familial aggregation of vitiligo. Archives of Dermatology. 1993;**129**(8):994-998

[4] Nath SK, Majumder PP, Nordlund JJ. Genetic epidemiology of vitiligo: Multilocus recessivity cross-validated. American Journal of Human Genetics. 1994;**55**(5):981-990

[5] Roberts GHL, Santorico SA, Spritz RA. Deep genotype imputation captures virtually all heritability of autoimmune vitiligo. Human Molecular Genetics. 2020;**29**(5):859-863. DOI: 10.1093/hmg/ddaa005

[6] Roberts GHL, Santorico SA, Spritz RA. The genetic architecture of vitiligo. Pigment Cell & Melanoma Research. 2020;**33**(1):8-15. DOI: 10.1111/pcmr.12848

[7] Spritz RA. The genetics of generalized vitiligo: Autoimmune pathways and an inverse relationship with malignant melanoma. Genome Medicine. 2010;**2**(10):78. DOI: 10.1186/gm199

[8] Shen C, Gao J, Sheng Y, Dou J, Zhou F, Zheng X, et al. Genetic susceptibility to vitiligo: GWAS approaches for identifying vitiligo susceptibility genes and loci. Frontiers in Genetics. 2016;**7**:3. DOI: 10.3389/fgene.2016.00003

[9] Jin Y, Andersen G, Yorgov D, Ferrara TM, Ben S, Brownson KM, et al. Genome-wide association studies of autoimmune vitiligo identify 23 new risk loci and highlight key pathways and regulatory variants. Nature Genetics. 2016;**48**(11):1418-1424. DOI: 10.1038/ng.3680

[10] Speeckaert R, Belpaire A, Speeckaert M, van Geel N. The delicate relation between melanocytes and skin immunity: A game of hide and seek. Pigment Cell & Melanoma Research. 2022;**35**:392-407. DOI: 10.1111/pcmr.13037

[11] Chang W-L, Ko C-H. The role of oxidative stress in vitiligo: An update on its pathogenesis and therapeutic implications. Cells. 2023;**12**(6):936. DOI: 10.3390/cells12060936

[12] Xie B, Song X. The impaired unfolded protein-premelanosome protein and transient receptor potential channels-autophagy axes in apoptotic melanocytes in vitiligo. Pigment Cell & Melanoma Research. 2022;**35**(1):6-17. DOI: 10.1111/pcmr.13006

[13] Chen J, Li S, Li C. Mechanisms of melanocyte death in vitiligo. Medicinal Research Reviews. 2021;**41**(2):1138-1166. DOI: 10.1002/med.21754

[14] Faraj S, Kemp EH, Gawkrodger DJ. Patho-immunological mechanisms of vitiligo: The role of the innate and adaptive immunities and environmental stress factors. Clinical and Experimental Immunology. 2022;**207**(1):27-43. DOI: 10.1093/cei/uxab002

[15] Marie J, Kovacs D, Pain C, Jouary T, Cota C, Vergier B, et al. Inflammasome activation and vitiligo/nonsegmental

vitiligo progression. The British Journal of Dermatology. 2014;**170**(4):816-823. DOI: 10.1111/bjd.12691

[16] Speeckaert R, Speeckaert M, De Schepper S, van Geel N. Biomarkers of disease activity in vitiligo: A systematic review. Autoimmunity Reviews. 2017;**16**(9):937-945. DOI: 10.1016/j.autrev.2017.07.005

[17] Tada M, Kohno M, Kasai S, Niwano Y. Generation mechanism of radical species by tyrosine-tyrosinase reaction. Journal of Clinical Biochemistry and Nutrition. 2010;**47**(2):162-166. DOI: 10.3164/jcbn.10-48

[18] Xuan Y, Yang Y, Xiang L, Zhang C. The role of oxidative stress in the pathogenesis of vitiligo: A culprit for melanocyte death. Oxidative Medicine and Cellular Longevity. 2022;**2022**:8498472. DOI: 10.1155/2022/8498472

[19] Pillaiyar T, Manickam M, Namasivayam V. Skin whitening agents: Medicinal chemistry perspective of tyrosinase inhibitors. Journal of Enzyme Inhibition and Medicinal Chemistry. 2017;**32**(1):403-425. DOI: 10.1080/14756366.2016.1256882

[20] Cameron MJ, Kelvin DJ. Cytokines, chemokines and their receptors. In: Madame Curie Bioscience Database [Internet]. Austin (TX): Landes Bioscience; 2000-2013. Available from: https://www.ncbi.nlm.nih.gov/books/NBK6294/

[21] Kany S, Vollrath JT, Relja B. Cytokines in inflammatory disease. International Journal of Molecular Sciences. 2019;**20**(23):6008. DOI: 10.3390/ijms20236008

[22] Zhao H, Wu L, Yan G, Chen Y, Zhou M, Wu Y, et al. Inflammation and tumor progression: Signaling pathways and targeted intervention. Signal Transduction and Targeted Therapy. 2021;**6**(1):263. DOI: 10.1038/s41392-021-00658-5

[23] Custurone P, Di Bartolomeo L, Irrera N, Borgia F, Altavilla D, Bitto A, et al. Role of cytokines in vitiligo: Pathogenesis and possible targets for old and new treatments. International Journal of Molecular Sciences. 2021;**22**(21):11429. DOI: 10.3390/ijms222111429

[24] Hariharan V, Klarquist J, Reust MJ, Koshoffer A, McKee MD, Boissy RE, et al. Monobenzyl ether of hydroquinone and 4-tertiary butyl phenol activate markedly different physiological responses in melanocytes: Relevance to skin depigmentation. The Journal of Investigative Dermatology. 2010;**130**(1):211-220. DOI: 10.1038/jid.2009.214

[25] Inoue S, Katayama I, Suzuki T, Tanemura A, Ito S, Abe Y, et al. Rhododendrol-induced leukoderma update II: Pathophysiology, mechanisms, risk evaluation, and possible mechanism-based treatments in comparison with vitiligo. The Journal of Dermatology. 2021;**48**:969-978. DOI: 10.1111/1346-8138.15878

[26] Harris JE. Chemical-induced vitiligo. Dermatologic Clinics. 2017;**35**(2):151-161. DOI: 10.1016/j.det.2016.11.006

[27] Marchioro HZ, Silva de Castro CC, Fava VM, Sakiyama PH, Dellatorre G, Miot HA. Update on the pathogenesis of vitiligo. Anais Brasileiros de Dermatologia. 2022;**97**(4):478-490. DOI: 10.1016/j.abd.2021.09.008

[28] Bharadwaj U, Kasembeli MM, Robinson P, Tweardy DJ. Targeting Janus kinases and signal transducer

and activator of transcription 3 to treat inflammation, fibrosis, and cancer: Rationale, progress, and caution. Pharmacological Reviews. 2020;**72**(2):486-526. DOI: 10.1124/pr.119.018440

[29] Kang C. Ruxolitinib cream 1.5%: A review in non-segmental vitiligo. Drugs. 2024;**84**(5):579-586. DOI: 10.1007/s40265-024-02027-2

[30] Pala V, Ribero S, Quaglino P, Mastorino L. Updates on potential therapeutic approaches for vitiligo: Janus kinase inhibitors and biologics. Journal of Clinical Medicine. 2023;**12**(23):7486. DOI: 10.3390/jcm12237486

# Section 3

# Alopecia

# Chapter 3

# Trichoscopy in the Diagnosis of Alopecia Areata

*Lidiya Todorova*

## Abstract

Alopecia areata (AA) is one of the most common hair loss disorders, with a prevalence of 0.1% - 0.2% of the general population. AA is regarded as a T-cell-mediated autoimmune condition characterized by non-scarring hair loss affecting only parts of the scalp, the entire scalp, or parts of the body. AA may manifest as a single episode or may have a relapsing course. Dermoscopy of the hair and scalp is known as trichoscopy. It is a useful method for diagnosing and monitoring hair and scalp disorders, as well as monitoring the effect of the applied treatment. The presence of exclamation mark hairs, black dots, triangular hairs, broken hairs, and pointed hairs in the alopecic patches indicates disease activity. One of the most common trichoscopic features of AA are the yellow dots - empty follicular openings filled with keratin and sebum. They predominate in long-standing, inactive diseases. Short vellus hairs are also common. The hair regrowth phase includes upright regrowing hairs and circle hairs. Diagnosis should be based on the coexistence of several trichoscopic findings rather than the presence of a single sign.

**Keywords:** alopecia, alopecia areata, hair loss, trichoscopy, dermoscopy, diagnosis, patchy hair loss, non-scarring, autoimmune hair loss

## 1. Introduction

Alopecia areata (AA) is one of the most common non-scarring hair loss disorders that have a prevalence of 0.1% - 0.2% in the general population. AA is considered an autoimmune T-cell-mediated condition and may manifest as a single episode or may have a relapsing course. It may affect only parts of the scalp with single (patchy alopecia or alopecia areata partialis) or multiple (alopecia areata reticularis) bald round hairless areas, the entire scalp (alopecia totalis), the entire scalp and bodily hairs (alopecia universalis), or only parts of the body. The diagnosis of AA is based on clinical examination and trichoscopy [1–7]. Dermoscopy of the hair and scalp is known as trichoscopy. It is a useful method for diagnosing and monitoring hair and scalp disorders, as well as monitoring the effect of the applied treatment. The diagnosis of AA should be based on the coexistence of several trichoscopic findings rather than the presence of a single sign. The trichoscopics markers such as exclamation mark hairs, black dots, triangular hairs, broken hairs, and pointed hairs in the alopecic patches indicate disease activity. One of the most common trichoscopic features of AA are the yellow dots - empty follicular openings filled with keratin and sebum.

**IntechOpen**

They predominate in long-standing, inactive diseases. Short vellus hairs are also common. Hair regrowth phase includes: upright regrowing hairs and circle hairs [1–7].

## 2. Trichoscopy

Dermoscopic examination of the hair and scalp is known as trichoscopy. The term was introduced by Lidia Rudnicka and Malgorzata Olszewska in 2006. Trichoscopy is a non-invasive method, a variation of dermatoscopy, in which the scalp and hair are examined with a standard dermatoscope (x10 magnification) or a digital videodermatoscope (x20–1000 magnification). It is a useful method in diagnosing and monitoring hair and scalp disorders, and in monitoring the effect of the treatment [1–7].

## 3. Trichoscopy in the diagnosis of alopecia areata

### 3.1 Trichoscopic markers in activity of alopecia areata

Trichoscopy is a useful tool in the diagnosis of AA and its management. Disease activity is characterized by black dots, exclamation mark hairs, triangular hairs, broken hairs, and pointed hairs in the alopecic patches. Black dots are pigmented hairs that are interrupted or destroyed at the scalp level. They correspond to remnants of hair shafts, which due to a disturbed anagen phase are broken before they emerge above the skin surface (**Figure 1**).

The most well-known trichoscopic feature of AA is the exclamation mark hairs (**Figure 2**). These are short hairs with a thick and dark distal end and a narrowed light proximal end. The hair shaft appears to be stuck into the follicular opening. These trichoscopic markers are result of the dystrophic mechanism of the hair condition. The presence of exclamation mark hairs at the borders of the alopecic areas indicates the activity of the disease [1–3, 9–11].

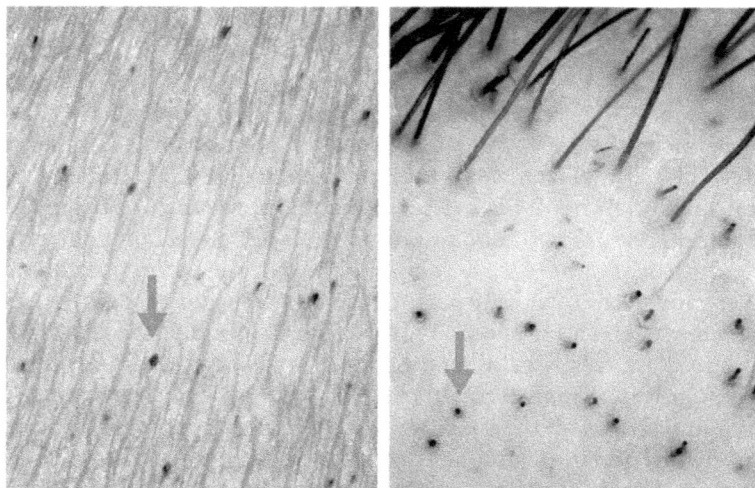

**Figure 1.**
*Black dots (Dino-Lite Edge AM7915MZT(R7) x70, images by Lidiya Todorova) [8].*

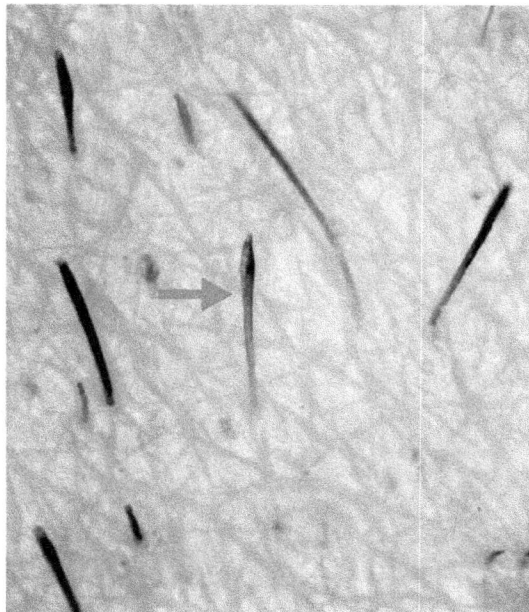

**Figure 2.**
*Exclamation mark hairs (Dino-Lite Edge AM7915MZT(R7) x70, image by Lidiya Todorova) [8].*

Other trichoscopic features of an active AA include a marker called triangular hairs. Those hairs have a distal pointed end and a proximal portion hidden by a whitish-gray veil. Presumably, like black dots, they are remnants of broken hairs, exclamation mark hairs, or tapered hairs [3, 10, 12–15].

Broken hairs are observed in 46% of patients. These are short hairs with normal hair shafts, but with irregular, choppy distal ends. They result from an irregular transverse breakage of the terminal hair shaft due to an inflammatory process or from rapid outgrowth of incompletely broken hairs that have previously formed black dots [3, 10, 12–15].

Tapered hairs are long exclamation mark hairs with the proximal end tapered and the distal end unable to be caught by the lens of the dermatoscope (**Figure 3**) [3, 10, 12–15].

Pohl-Pincus constrictions are areas of reduced hair thickness of the hair shaft. These constrictions occur most commonly when the metabolic and mitotic activity of hair follicles is rapidly and repeatedly suppressed [3, 10, 12–16].

Normal-appearing hairs that can easily break when bent or pressed have also been described in AA. This phenomenon is called "coudability," meaning "elbow effect" [17]. These "coudability hairs" are also associated with AA activity [13] (**Table 1**).

## 3.2 Trichoscopic markers in chronic alopecia areata

Another common trichoscopic sign of AA is the yellow dots (**Figure 4**). This finding predominates in long-standing, and inactive diseases. The yellow dots represent empty follicular openings filled with keratin and sebum. In AA, they appear in groups reflecting the number of hairs in the follicular units. This marker can also be present in the acute form of AA.

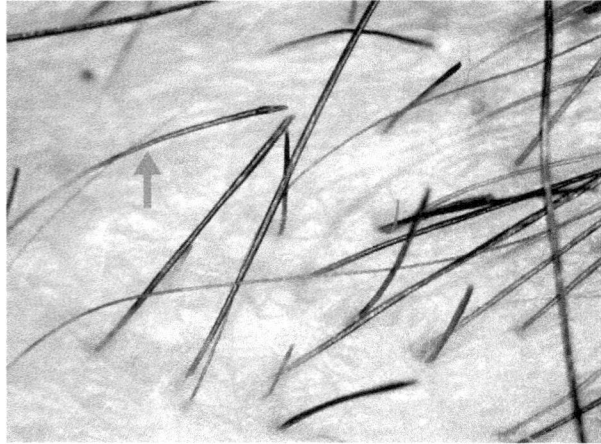

**Figure 3.**
*Tapered hairs (Dino-Lite Edge AM7915MZT(R7) x70, image by Lidiya Todorova) [8].*

| Trichoscopic sign | Description |
|---|---|
| Exclamation mark hair | They are formed as a result of the growth of broken hair shafts and are characterized by a distal, irregularly broken end that is wider than the proximal part of the hair shaft. |
| Black dots or cadaverized hairs | Correspond to remnants of hair shafts, which, due to an anagenic phase disturbance, are broken before they emerge above the skin surface. |
| Triangular hairs or short hidden hairs) | They have a distal pointed end and a proximal part hidden by a whitish-gray veil. They are seen more commonly in patients with active hair loss. Presumed to be like black dots, they are considered remnants of broken hairs, exclamation mark-type hairs, or pointed hairs. |
| Broken hairs | These are short hairs with hair shafts that appear normal except for irregular, ragged distal ends. Broken hairs result from an irregular transverse breakage of the terminal hair shaft due to an inflammatory process or from rapid regrowth of incompletely broken hairs that have previously formed black dots. |
| Tapered hairs | These are very long exclamation mark hairs. Their proximal end is narrowed and the distal end cannot be covered by the lens of the dermatscope. |
| "Coudability hairs" | Normal-looking hairs that bend easily when pressed or pushed. |
| Pohl-Pincus constrictions | The term refers to areas of reduced hair thickness but within the hair shaft. These constrictions occur most commonly when the metabolic and mitotic activity of the hair follicle is rapidly and repeatedly suppressed. |
| Yellow dots | They are round or polycyclic, yellow or yellowish-red dots of various sizes, evenly distributed in the affected area, corresponding to dilated and slightly thickened follicular orifices filled with horny matter and sebum, with or without hair shafts within them. They are considered the most characteristic finding in alopecia partialis and are seen in 95% of patients with phototype I-IV and in 40–60% of patients with phototype V-VI skin. |
| Short vellus hairs | Short newly grown and vellus hairs less than 10 mm in length. They represent hairs that are unable to continue their anagen growth. They may be white in color and seen in groups. |
| Upright regrowing hairs | New, healthy, regrowing hairs that have a pointed end and an upright position. |

| Trichoscopic sign | Description |
|---|---|
| Pigtail hairs or circle hairs | Pigtail hairs are short, regrowing, properly curled hairs that have pointed ends. This is a rare finding associated with hair growth in patients with acute hair loss. |
| Coiled hairs | These hairs are distinguished from pigtail hairs by their irregular texture and choppy distal end. |
| White dots | Associated with the development of fibrosis in long hair loss. |

**Table 1.**
*Description of trichoscopic signs in AA [3, 7, 8, 10, 18].*

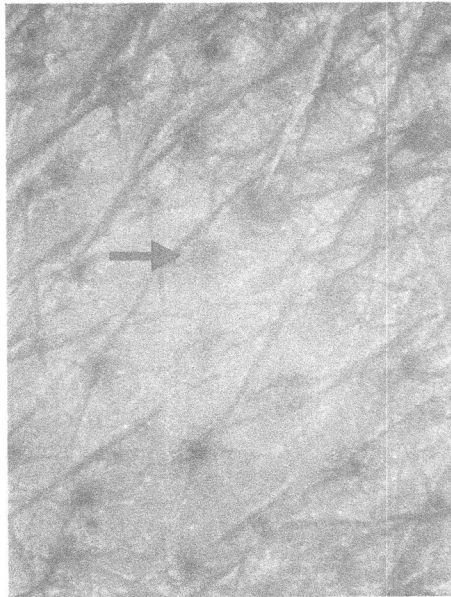

**Figure 4.**
*Yellow dots (Dino-Lite Edge AM7915MZT(R7) x70, image by Lidiya Todorova) [8].*

Short vellus hairs and unpigmented hair shafts less than 10 mm in length and less than 0.03 mm in thickness are also common (**Figure 5**). Short vellus hairs are less than 10 mm long. They represent hairs that are unable to continue their anagen growth (**Table 1**) [1–7, 9, 10, 16].

## 3.3 Trichoscopic markers in hair growth phase in alopecia areata

Hair recovery in AA can be monitored with trichoscopy. The main markers include upright regrowing hairs that are anagen hairs, which are pointed and grow in an upright position); coiled hairs, which are uniformly curved in their distal part. Pigtail hairs are short, growing, properly curled, and have pointed ends. This is a rare finding associated with hair growth in patients with acute hair loss. Coiled hairs are differentiated from pigtail hairs by their irregular texture and choppy distal end (**Table 1**) [3, 10, 15, 16].

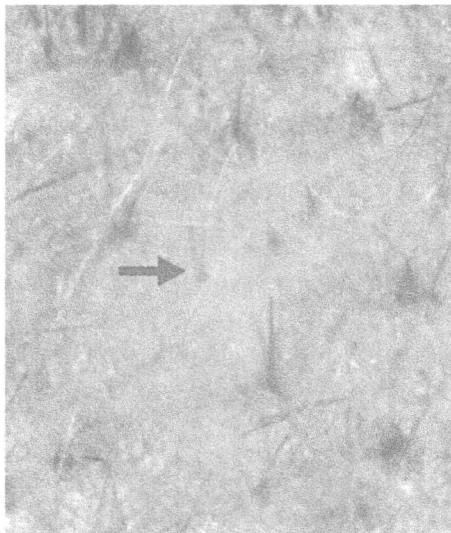

**Figure 5.**
*Vellus hairs (Dino-Lite Edge AM7915MZT(R7) x70, image by Lidiya Todorova) [8].*

## 3.4 Other trichoscopic markers in alopecia areata

There are also other interesting trichoscopic signs that have been associated with alopecia areata but are less frequent. The honeycomb pattern consists of grouped and homogeneously colored brown oval spots. It is observed in chronic sun exposed areas and in dark-skinned individuals [7, 8, 18–21].

Dirty dots are non-microbial particles from the environment and are easily removed after shampooing. They may be brown, black, red, yellow or blue, and may look like fibers [3, 7, 8, 18–21].

There are two types of white dots described: large and small. The large white dots occur in chronic AA and correspond to areas of follicular fibrosis. Smaller white dots correspond to the openings of eccrine sweat glands [3, 7, 8, 18–21].

Tulip hairs are leaf-shaped hairs with hyperpigmentation at the distal end (**Figure 6**) [3, 4, 8, 10].

## 3.5 Assessing disease activity, severity, duration and type of alopecia areata with trichosopy

Trichoscopy is a useful tool in assessing not only disease activity, but also severity and duration. More precisely, severe active AA is characterized by the presence of black dots, yellow dots, reduced amount of vellus hairs, honeycomb pattern, and clusters of white dots. In the mild active AA there are only exclamation mark hairs. Acute AA has the presence of exclamation mark hairs, black dots, and vellus hairs, while chronic AA features yellow dots, smooth and fine hair on the scalp and very weak growth of pigmented hairs inhomogeneous distribution (**Table 2**) [3].

There are different types of the condition, ranging from small single alopecic patches to the absence of all hairs on the body. It is described that AA incognita features extensive amount of pigtail hair (57.9%), newly growing hairs, black dots, yellow

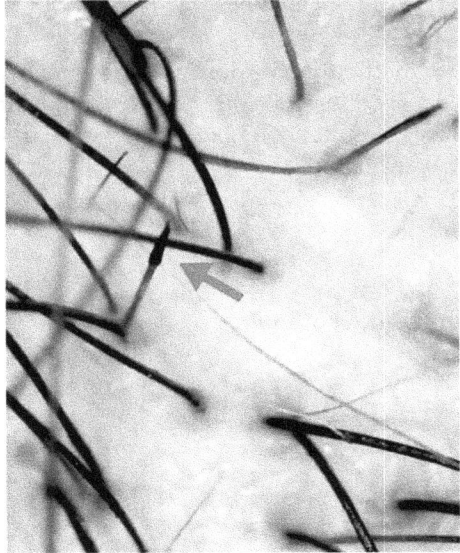

**Figure 6.**
*Tulip hairs (Dino-Lite Edge AM7915MZT(R7) x70, image by Lidiya Todorova) [8].*

dots distributed diffusely, mainly affecting the occipital and parietal region, and proportionally to the severity of the hair loss. In AA diffusa, the inflammatory damage to the follicles is much greater than in AA incognita. There is a greater presence of dystrophic hairs, black dots (36%), and yellow dots in the parietal and anterior-temporal areas of the scalp. In the ophiasis AA, the trichoscopy shows mainly black dots, but there are no yellow dots. Positive prognostic markers for alopecia totalis and universalis include pigmented vellus hairs and upright regrowing hairs [3, 8].

| Activity of AA | Activity of AA | • Exclamation mark hairs |
| --- | --- | --- |
| | | • Black dots |
| | | • Pointed hairs |
| | | • Tapered hairs |
| | | • Broken hairs |
| | | • *Pohl-Pinkus* constrictions |
| | | • Coudability hairs |
| | | • Yellow dots |
| | Chronic AA | • Yellow dots |
| | | • Vellus hairs |
| | Hair growth in AA | • Upright regrowing hairs |
| | | • Pigtail hairs |
| | | • Circle hairs |
| | | • Vellus hairs |

**Table 2.**
*Trichoscopy based on activity and duration of alopecia areata.*

## 4. Conclusion

Trichoscopy is a useful method to diagnose and monitor AA. The diagnosis of AA should be based on clinical examination and trichoscopy. The trichoscopic evaluation should take into account the simultaneous existence of several trichoscopic findings rather than the presence of a single sign.

## Conflict of interest

The author declares no conflict of interest.

## Author details

Lidiya Todorova
Dermatology and Venereology Department, Medical University – Plovdiv, Plovdiv, Bulgaria

*Address all correspondence to: lidiatodorova@gmail.com

IntechOpen

# References

[1] Todorova LN, Abadjieva TI. Platelet-rich plasma in alopecia areata: A case report with a mini review of literature. Cureus. 2023;**15**(5):e38751. DOI: 10.7759/cureus.38751

[2] Abadjieva TI, Todorova LN, Gardjeva PA, Murdjeva MA. Platelet-rich plasma efficacy in alopecia areata patients with normal and elevated levels of antibodies against thyroglobulin and thyroid peroxidase. Folia Medica (Plovdiv). 2024;**66**(1):66-72. DOI: 10.3897/folmed.66.e115484

[3] Gómez-Quispe H et al. Trichoscopy in alopecia Areata. Actas Dermo-Sifiliográficas. 2023;**114**(1):25-32. DOI: 10.1016/j.ad.2022.08.018

[4] Miteva M, Tosti A. Hair and scalp dermatoscopy. Journal of the American Academy of Dermatology. 2012;**67**(5):1040-1048. DOI: 10.1016/j.jaad.2012.02.013

[5] Olszewska M et al. Trichoscopy. Archives of Dermatology. 2008;**144**:8. DOI: 10.1001/archderm.144.8.1007

[6] Rudnicka L et al. Presence and future of dermoscopy [meeting report]. Expert Review of Dermatology. 2006;**1**(6):769-772. DOI: 10.1586/17469872.1.6.769

[7] Waśkiel-Burnat A et al. Trichoscopy of alopecia areata in children. A retrospective comparative analysis of 50 children and 50 adults. Pediatric Dermatology. 2019;**36**(5):640-645. DOI: 10.1111/pde.13912

[8] Todorova LN. Clinical and Therapeutic Studies in Alopecia Areata [Thesis]. Plovdiv: Medical University – Plovdiv; 2024

[9] Lacarrubba F et al. Videodermatoscopy enhances diagnostic capability in some forms of hair loss. American Journal of Clinical Dermatology. 2004;**5**(3):205-208. DOI: 10.2165/00128071-200405030-00009

[10] Rudnicka L et al. Atlas of Trichoscopy: Dermoscopy in Hair and Scalp Disease. London: Springer; 2012. DOI: 10.1007/978-1-4471-4486-1

[11] Rudnicka L et al. Hair shafts in Trichoscopy. Dermatologic Clinics. 2013;**31**(4):695-708. DOI: 10.1016/j.det.2013.06.007

[12] Guttikonda AS et al. Evaluation of clinical significance of Dermoscopy in alopecia Areata. Indian Journal of Dermatology. 2016;**61**(6):628-633. DOI: 10.4103/0019-5154.193668

[13] Inui S et al. Clinical significance of dermoscopy in alopecia areata: Analysis of 300 cases. International Journal of Dermatology. 2008;**47**(7):688-693. DOI: 10.1111/j.1365-4632.2008.03692.x

[14] Rudnicka L et al. Trichoscopy update 2011. Journal of Dermatological Case Reports. 2011;**5**(4):828-828. DOI: 10.3315/jdcr.2011.1083

[15] Waśkiel-Burnat A et al. Alopecia areata predictive score: A new trichoscopy-based tool to predict treatment outcome in patients with patchy alopecia areata. Journal of Cosmetic Dermatology. 2020;**19**(3):746-751. DOI: 10.1111/jocd.13064

[16] Waśkiel A et al. Trichoscopy of alopecia areata: An update. The Journal of Dermatology. 2018;**45**(6):692-700. DOI: 10.1111/1346-8138.14283

[17] Shuster S. "Coudability": A new physical sign of alopecia areata. The British Journal of Dermatology. 1984;**111**(5):629-629

[18] Dobrev H. Application of trichoscopy in clinical practice. Health.bg. 2013;**9**:34-37 [ISSN 1314-2569] [In Bulgarian]

[19] Meah N et al. The alopecia Areata consensus of experts (ACE) study: Results of an international expert opinion on treatments for alopecia areata. Journal of the American Academy of Dermatology. 2020;**83**(1):123-130. DOI: 10.1016/j.jaad.2020.03.004

[20] Rakowska A et al. Alopecia areata. Diagnostic and therapeutic recommendations of the polish dermatological society. Part 1. Diagnosis and severity assessment. Dermatology Review/Przegląd Dermatologiczny. 2023;**110**(2):89-100. DOI: 10.5114/dr.2023.127704

[21] Rakowska A et al. Alopecia areata. Diagnostic and therapeutic recommendations of the polish Society of Dermatology. Part 2: Treatment. Dermatology Review/Przegląd Dermatologiczny. 2023;**110**(2):101-120. DOI: 10.5114/dr.2023.127705

Section 4

# Systemic Sclerosis

Chapter 4

# Systemic Scleroderma: Orofacial Manifestations and Therapeutic Approaches

*Ghada Bouslama, Aya Mtiri, Nour Sayda Ben Messaoud, Lamia Oualha and Souha Ben Youssef*

## Abstract

Systemic scleroderma, a multifaceted autoimmune disease, often presents with significant orofacial manifestations that pose substantial challenges in clinical management. This chapter provides a comprehensive review of the various orofacial complications associated with systemic scleroderma, including microstomia, xerostomia, periodontal disease, and temporomandibular joint disorders. The pathophysiological mechanisms underlying these manifestations are explored, highlighting the importance of early recognition and intervention. Additionally, this chapter discusses current therapeutic approaches, emphasizing the need for a multidisciplinary strategy that encompasses physical therapy, surgical options and prosthetic rehabilitation. This review aims to enhance understanding among healthcare professionals and improve patient outcomes through a more informed and integrated approach to care.

**Keywords:** systemic sclerosis, oral manifestation, microstomia, hyposalivation, treatment

## 1. Introduction

Systemic sclerosis (SSc) is an autoimmune disease belonging to the family of connective tissue diseases, predominantly affecting women. Characterized by fibrosis, it results from the simultaneous involvement of the immune system, vascular system, and connective tissue. The life expectancy of patients is variable and primarily depends on numerous visceral complications, particularly affecting the heart, lungs, and digestive system [1, 2].

Systemic sclerosis is present in various forms, ranging from localized scleroderma to overlap syndromes, where scleroderma signs are associated with Sjögren's syndrome, systemic lupus erythematosus, rheumatoid arthritis, dermato- or polymyositis, or early mixed connective tissue disease [3].

IntechOpen

This autoimmune disease is characterized by severe fibrosis. The skin, blood vessels, muscles, and internal organs can be affected to varying degrees, including the orofacial region.

The aim of this chapter is to highlight the different orodental and facial manifestations of systemic sclerosis and to describe the specific management modalities for these patients.

## 2. Pathophysiology

Although the pathophysiology of SSc remains unclear, it appears to result from the combined dysfunction of endothelial cells, lymphocytes, and fibroblasts. These abnormalities lead to the activation of fibroblasts and subsequent fibrosis [2, 4].

Regarding vascular abnormalities, the primary lesion occurs at the level of the vascular endothelium including capillaries, small arteries, and arterioles, and may be due to anti-endothelial cell antibodies frequently found in patients with SSc. This apoptotic phenomenon precedes clinical signs as well as lymphocyte cell infiltration in the dermis [5].

Fibroblast abnormalities results from an uncontrolled synthesis of extracellular matrix (ECM) proteins through several mechanisms: TGF-$\beta$ is excessively synthesized by endothelial cells, lymphocytes, and fibroblasts, leading to their proliferation and phenotypic differentiation into myofibroblasts [6, 7].

Considering the immune dysregulation, it results from the activation of B lymphocytes (LB), which explains the presence of antinuclear antibodies in the serum of the majority (90%) of patients with scleroderma, notably including anti-topoisomerase I antibodies and anti-centromere antibodies [6, 8].

## 3. Clinical manifestations of systemic sclerosis

### 3.1 General manifestations

#### 3.1.1 Cutaneous manifestations

Raynaud's phenomenon is observed in nearly all patients (95%). It is often the first clinical sign of the disease, and its detection plays a major role in early diagnosis. This phenomenon is initially triggered by cold or stress, causing the skin to turn white initially, then blue due to cyanosis, and finally red accompanied by hyperemia [8–10].

Cutaneous sclerosis is also characteristic of the disease. The Rodnan skin score (a measure of skin thickness) is generally used to quantify the skin involvement and progression of lesions. It can affect the limbs, back, abdomen and face. The Scoring of each individual cutaneous area vary from "0" for normal skin to "3" for severe skin thickness [11].

Initially, the fingers are affected (sclerodactyly), and then the sclerosis extends to the metacarpophalangeal joints, leading to a loss of wrist mobility. This sclerodactyly significantly decreases the quality of life of these patients, particularly hindering oral hygiene practices (**Figure 1**) [9].

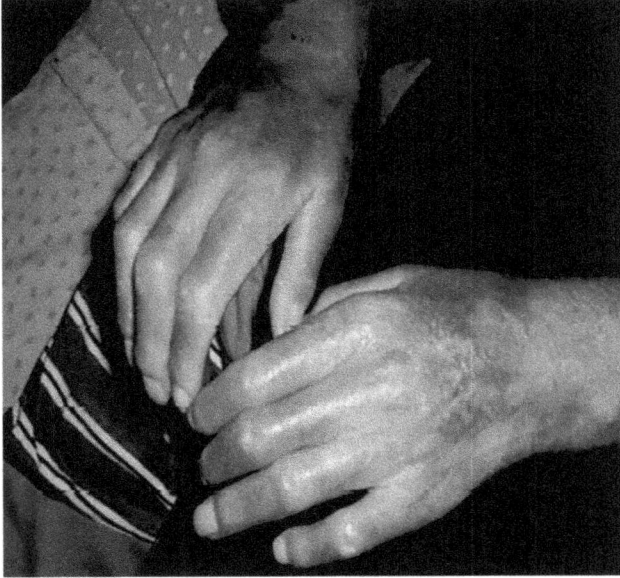

**Figure 1.**
*Cutaneous sclerosis affecting the fingers (sclerodactyly).*

### 3.1.2 Visceral manifestations

Visceral symptoms are frequent, presenting from the onset of the disease or appearing during its progression [8, 9, 12]. They include:

1. Digestive involvement in 80% of cases with esophageal-gastro-intestinal dyskinesia.

2. Pulmonary involvement, including fibrosing interstitial pneumonitis and pulmonary arterial hypertension.

3. Cardiac involvement, which can be primary due to the sclerodermic process, could manifest as cardiomyopathy, pericarditis, conduction disturbances, and/or arrhythmias, or secondary to pulmonary or renal lesions.

4. Renal involvement, which is one of the leading causes of death.

### 3.1.3 Articular and muscular manifestations

These are present in 40–90% of cases, manifesting as chronic polyarthralgia or acroparesthesia, myopathy, or myasthenia [9].

Other possible manifestations include trigeminal neuralgia, vasculitis, polyneuropathy, or ocular involvement. Hepatic involvement is authenticated in only 10% of cases [13, 14].

## 3.2 Facial and oro-dental manifestations

The orofacial manifestations of systemic sclerosis are numerous but often under-diagnosed due to the presence of more severe systemic complications [15].

### 3.2.1 Facial manifestations

Clinical manifestations are numerous and appear early. They lead to a characteristic "mask-like" face. Cutaneous fibrosis causes the facial skin sclerosis, thinning of the lips, disappearance of skin wrinkles, a pointed nose, and the development of vertical furrows around the mouth [15, 16]. Telangiectasias due to vasospasms of small vessels appear on the cheeks, lips, or nose. Microstomia and microcheilia, due to the fibrosis of soft tissues, can affect the patient's social life and hinder mandibular movements (**Figure 2**).

### 3.2.2 Mucosal and secretory manifestations

Collagenous changes make the mucosa thin, pale, sclerotic, and sometimes ulcerated. Telangiectasias can be observed. The fibrotic process affects the tongue, soft palate, and pharynx, potentially leading to dysphagia, dysgeusia, or stomatodynia. Shortening and loss of elasticity of the lingual frenulum decrease tongue mobility, making speech and swallowing difficult [11, 12, 15].

Gastroesophageal reflux disease (GERD) resulting from digestive involvement can cause demineralization of the dental surface, even in the presence of saliva. This decrease in oral pH is exacerbated by xerostomia. One-quarter of patients with GERD exhibit dental erosions, primarily located on the palatal surfaces of maxillary teeth. An erythema may also be present on the palatal mucosa.

Xerostomia is reported by the majority of patients, leading to an increased risk of caries due to the reduced effectiveness of saliva against cariogenic bacteria and oral Candida infections. In most cases, xerostomia in scleroderma patients is due to fibrosis of the capillaries and excretory ducts of the salivary glands. However, Sjögren's syndrome, responsible for dry mouth due to lymphocytic infiltration of the salivary glands, can also be present as part of an overlap syndrome [15, 16].

### 3.2.3 Periodontal and dental manifestations

Clinically, periodontal involvement manifests as a higher number of missing teeth, attachment loss, bleeding on probing, and increased probing depth. These issues are primarily due to microstomia, cutaneous and articular involvement, leading to poor oral hygiene.

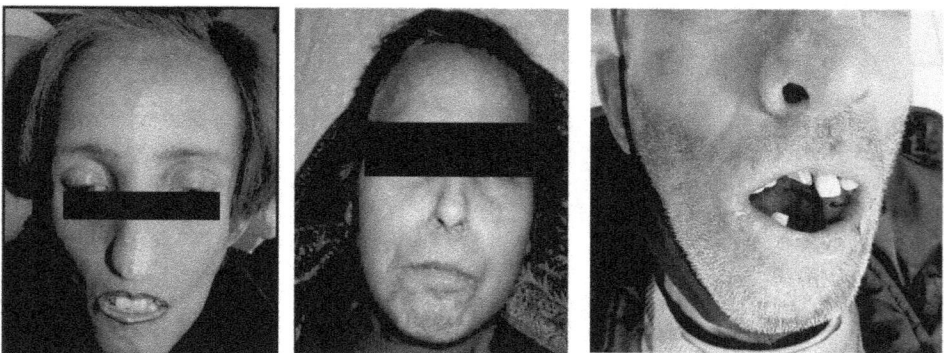

**Figure 2.**
*Facial characteristics of patients with scleroderma: telangiectasias, lip thinning, microstomia.*

Radiographically, a characteristic feature of SSc is the widening of the periodontal ligament, without consequences on tooth mobility and not associated with periodontitis. This thickening, visible in the early stages of the disease, is likely due to collagen overproduction. Additionally, thickening of the alveolar bone's lamina dura is noticed, primarily in the posterior teeth (**Figure 3**) [11, 15, 17].

### 3.2.4 Bone and articular manifestations

A phenomenon of bone resorption can affect the mandibular arch, preferentially the mandibular angle, condyle, or coronoid process in patients with a diffuse form of SSc. The origin is ischemic, due to microvasculopathy, and also due to pressure secondary to skin and muscle atrophy. In some cases, significant resorption can cause

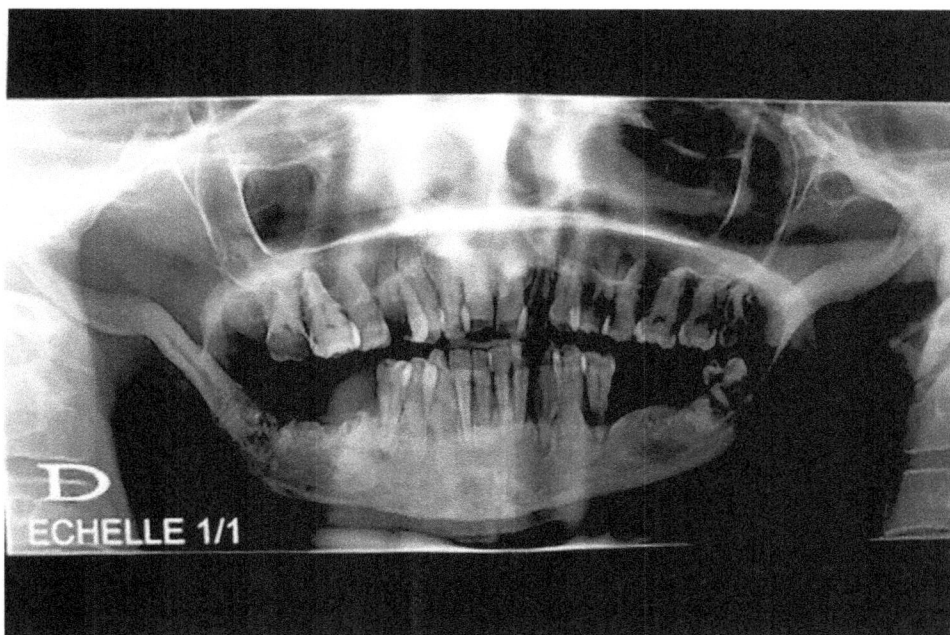

**Figure 3.**
*Panoramic radiograph showing periodontal ligament widening.*

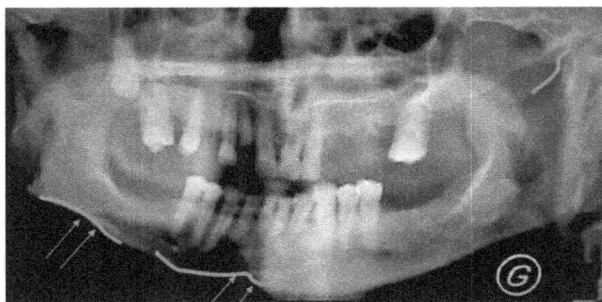

**Figure 4.**
*Bone resorption at the level of the left condyle, the right basilar border, and the right mandibular angle.*

compression of the inferior alveolar nerve and trigeminal neuropathies, or even a pathological fracture of the mandible [12, 15].

Temporomandibular joint (TMJ) disorders are also observed due to bone resorption, especially when it occurs at the articular surfaces. Symptoms of masticatory apparatus dysfunction (noise, pain, dyskinesia) correlate with the duration of the disease. Generally, TMJ disorders related to systemic sclerosis are poorly documented (**Figure 4**) [18].

## 4. Management of oral and dental complications related to systemic sclerosis

### 4.1 Cutaneous and mucosal aspects

*4.1.1 Management of xerostomia (dry mouth)*

Management strategies include recommendations for alleviating discomfort with simple oral lubricants, saliva substitutes, salivary stimulants, and intraoral stimulation [15, 17–20].

- *Oral lubricants*: Regular hydration is essential. From a dietary perspective, it is advisable to avoid spicy or acidic foods, prefer olive oil or milk, which have lubricating and remineralizing properties.

- *Saliva substitutes*: These are available in various forms, including gels, toothpastes, liquids, aerosols, or mouth rinses, and possess antimicrobial, remineralizing, or buffering properties similar to saliva. Regardless of their composition, available saliva substitutes provide only short-term relief, require frequent renewal, and do not offer sustained symptom relief [19, 20].

- *Salivary stimulants*: These include parasympathomimetic sialogogues such as pilocarpine and cevimeline. The effects typically manifest 30 minutes after administration and last for 3–4 hours. Common side effects include excessive sweating, which can reduce adherence to treatment. Both drugs are contraindicated in patients with pulmonary or cardiovascular diseases [15, 19, 20].

*4.1.2 Management of mucosal and gingival lesions*

The presence of a removable prosthesis combined with xerostomia frequently leads to mucosal pain. It is recommended to use an antiseptic oral gel containing chlorhexidine. If the use of the prosthesis results in the development of an ulcer, the occlusion and peripheral seals should be checked and adjusted. Application of a topical anesthetic containing 2% lidocaine can provide relief to the patient [19].

*4.1.3 Management of oral candidiasis infections*

The occurrence of oral candidiasis in patients with scleroderma is favored by extrinsic factors (such as the use of broad-spectrum antibiotics, antiseptics, corticosteroids, or immunosuppressants) and intrinsic factors (xerostomia) [21, 22] (**Figure 5**). The infection may manifest in different forms:

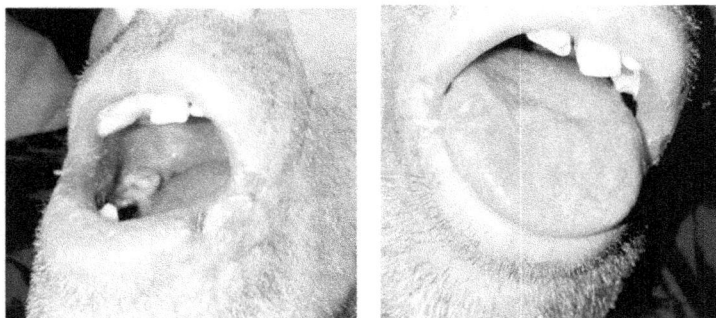

**Figure 5.**
*Clinical manifestations of chronic erythematous candidosis.*

- Pseudomembranous candidiasis

- Chronic erythematous candidiasis

- Denture stomatitis

In daily practice, if antibiotic treatment for prophylactic or curative purposes is indicated for a scleroderma patient with xerostomia, the choice of antibiotic should be considered carefully, as broad-spectrum antibiotics may induce candidiasis.

If fungal infection is confirmed, initial treatment should be local such as nystatin, amphotericin B in an oral solution, or miconazole gel applied for 2–3 weeks. Local treatment should be maintained in contact with the mucosa for as long as possible, preferably outside of meal and drink times. The use of a prosthesis should be avoided throughout the topical treatment period to ensure that the medication reaches all tissues.

In cases of local treatment failure, systemic antifungal therapy should be continued with azoles: fluconazole or itraconazole for 2 weeks [21, 22]. In all cases, it is crucial to address existing hyposalivation with a patient-appropriate therapeutic approach.

## 4.2 Dental and periodontal aspects

### 4.2.1 Adapted oral hygiene

Sclerodactyly decreases manual dexterity, which poses a challenge for maintaining good oral hygiene. The use of an electric toothbrush can improve hygiene in these patients 15. A pediatric toothbrush may be useful for cleaning hard-to-reach areas. Interdental jet devices can also be employed when digital ulcers or Raynaud's phenomenon limit manual interdental cleaning [22].

### 4.2.2 Prevention and treatment of dental caries

The prevention of dental caries in scleroderma patients, and more generally in patients with hyposalivation, involves several steps [21, 22].

- Improving salivary flow with appropriate therapy.

- Reducing the number of cariogenic bacteria in the oral cavity through regular use of chlorhexidine.

- Implementing dietary modifications to minimize carbohydrate intake.

These measures should be combined with good oral hygiene and regular visits to the dentist [23].

### 4.2.3 Treatment of periodontal disease

Treatment follows the standard periodontal therapy protocol:

- Oral hygiene education

- Scaling and root planing

- Radiographic evaluation: panoramic X-ray and periapical status

- Periodontal probing

- Reevaluation and maintenance

*Infectious risk*: The use of corticosteroids at a dosage >10 mg per day (equivalent to prednisone) or ≤1 mg/kg/day for more than 8 days, as well as immunosuppressive therapy, increases the scleroderma patient's risk of infection compared to the general population 25. If scaling or root planing is required, antibiotic prophylaxis may be considered. As with the general population, curative antibiotic therapy is recommended for localized or generalized aggressive periodontitis [24, 25].

## 4.3 Articular and skeletal aspects

### 4.3.1 Management of microstomia

Mouth opening limitation is considered severe when the interincisal distance is less than 30 mm. While surgical interventions such as bilateral commissurotomy or commissuroplasty exist, they are often considered too invasive [15]. Non-surgical alternatives, which are simpler and should be implemented at the early stages of the disease, can be proposed to increase mouth opening and skin elasticity. These include perioral muscle reeducation exercises.

The TheraBite Jaw Motion Rehabilitation System® is a medical device designed to address mandibular hypomobility. By facilitating repetitive and passive movements controlled directly by the patient, it helps restore mobility and flexibility of the mandibular musculature, joints, and connective tissue (**Figure 6**) [15].

Additionally, therapies involving the injection of autologous fat and adipose-derived stromal cells into the perioral region have been described, resulting in improved mouth opening and oral function. Facial esthetics and the Rodman score are also enhanced [26].

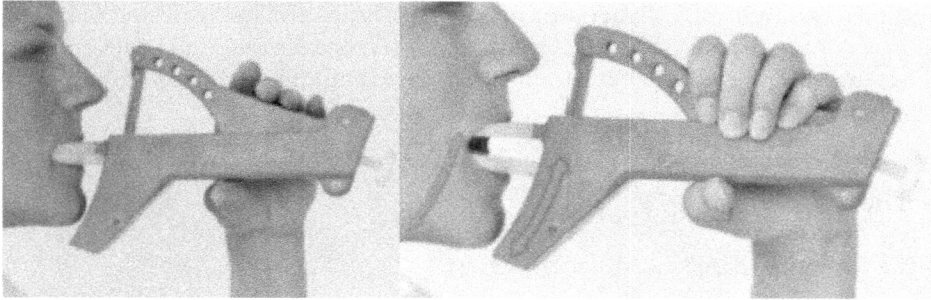

**Figure 6.**
*Medical device therabite jaw motion rehabilitation system [26].*

Platelet-Rich Fibrin (PRF) also shows promise as an effective approach for treating refractory cutaneous ulcers in systemic sclerosis, as well as for addressing minor facial wrinkles. However, additional scientific based evidence is needed to conclusively demonstrate PRF's role in wound healing and its pain-reducing properties in sclero-dermic skin ulcers [27].

### 4.3.2 Management of bone resorption

Bone resorption is typically asymptomatic and is often discovered incidentally during panoramic radiography. It generally does not require treatment; however, monitoring is necessary since there is a risk of pathological mandibular fracture. In cases of advanced condylar destruction, condylectomy and replacement of the condyles with chondrocostal grafts are viable options, yielding stable and functional long-term results [15, 23].

### 4.3.3 Management of articular pain

Mild arthralgias affecting the joints, including the temporomandibular joint (TMJ), are generally well managed with non-steroidal anti-inflammatory drugs (NSAIDs), disease-modifying antirheumatic drugs (DMARDs) such as hydroxychlo-roquine, or low-dose systemic corticosteroids (7.5 mg/day). For more severe arthral-gias, methotrexate may be used [4].

## 5. Conclusion

Given the clinical and radiological buccal-facial aspects of systemic sclerosis, early diagnosis could be achieved at the initial stage of the disease, often allowing treatment to be more effective. Close collaboration between the dentist, dermatologist, rheumatologist, and internist is essential to ensure monitoring of this disease, which can have a very severe progression.

Systemic scleroderma is a complex autoimmune disorder that significantly impacts the orofacial region, presenting challenges in both diagnosis and management. The orofacial manifestations, including microstomia, xerostomia, and periodontal disease, need a comprehensive, multidisciplinary therapeutic approach to improve patient outcomes. Early intervention and tailored treatment plans are crucial.

Continued research and collaboration among healthcare professionals, including dentists, dermatologists, rheumatologists, and internists are essential to advance our understanding and enhance the quality of care for individuals with systemic scleroderma.

## Conflict of interest

The authors declare no conflict of interest.

## Author details

Ghada Bouslama*, Aya Mtiri, Nour Sayda Ben Messaoud, Lamia Oualha and Souha Ben Youssef
Dentistry Department, Research Laboratory LR 12SP10: Functional and Aesthetic Rehabilitation of Maxillary, Farhat Hached Hospital, University of Sousse, Sousse, Tunisia

*Address all correspondence to: bouslama.ghada@yahoo.fr

## IntechOpen

# References

[1] Swynghedauw B. Sclérodermie. Archives des Maladies du Coeur et des Vaisseaux - Pratique. 2009;**2009**(179):35-36

[2] Puzenat E, Aubin F, Humbert P. Sclérodermie systémique. EMC-Dermatologie. 2009;**5**(1):1-14

[3] Cabane J. Critères de classification des sclérodermies. Presse Médicale. 2006;**35**(12, Part 2):1916-1922

[4] Bessis D, Francès C, Guillot B, Guilhou J-J. Manifestations dermatologiques des connectivites, vasculites et affections systémiques apparentées. Paris Berlin Heidelberg: Springer; 2006 (Dermatologie et médecine)

[5] Yamamoto T. Autoimmune mechanisms of scleroderma and a role of oxidative stress. Self/Nonself. 2011;**2**(1):4-10

[6] Servettaz A, Agard C, Tamby MC, Guilpain P, Guillevin L, Mouthon L. Physiopathologie de la sclérodermie systémique: état des lieux sur une affection aux multiples facettes. Presse Médicale. 2006;**35**(12, Part 2):1903-1915

[7] Mouthon L. Sclérodermie systémique: de la physiopathologie au traitement. Rev Médecine Interne. 2007;**28**:S266-S272

[8] Allanore Y, Avouac J, Kahan A. Systemic sclerosis: An update in 2008. Joint, Bone, Spine. 2008;**75**(6):650-655

[9] Sticherling M. Systemic sclerosis – Dermatological aspects. Part 1: Pathogenesis, epidemiology, clinical findings. JDDG. Journal der Deutschen Dermatologischen Gesellschaft. 2012;**10**(10):705-716

[10] Bongi SM, Rosso AD, Miniati I, Galluccio F, Landi G, Tai G, et al. The Italian version of the Mouth Handicap in Systemic Sclerosis scale (MHISS) is valid, reliable and useful in assessing oral health-related quality of life (OHRQoL) in systemic sclerosis (SSc) patients. Rheumatology International. 2012;**32**(9):2785-2790

[11] Khanna D et al. Standardization of the modified Rodnan skin score for use in clinical trials of systemic sclerosis. Journal of Scleroderma and Related Disorders. 2017;**2**(1):11-18

[12] Mouthon L. L'atteinte de la main dans la sclérodermie systémique. Presse Médicale. 2013;**42**(12):1616-1626

[13] Jung S, Martin T, Schmittbuhl M, Huck O. The spectrum of orofacial manifestations in systemic sclerosis: A challenging management. Oral Diseases. 2017;**23**(4):424-439

[14] Isola G, Williams RC, Gullo AL, Ramaglia L, Matarese M, Iorio-Siciliano V, et al. Risk association between scleroderma disease characteristics, periodontitis, and tooth loss. Clinical Rheumatology. 2017;**36**(12):2733-2741

[15] Crincoli V, Fatone L, Fanelli M, Rotolo RP, Chialà A, Favia G, et al. Orofacial manifestations and temporomandibular disorders of systemic scleroderma: An observational study. International Journal of Molecular Sciences. 2016;**17**(7):1189

[16] Isola G et al. Risk association between scleroderma disease characteristics, periodontitis, and tooth loss. Clinical Rheumatology. 2017;**36**:2733-2741

[17] Baron M, Hudson M, Tatibouet S, Steele R, Lo E, Gravel S, et al. The Canadian systemic sclerosis oral health study: Orofacial manifestations and oral health-related quality of life in systemic sclerosis compared with the general population. Rheumatology (Oxford, England). 2014;**53**(8):1386-1394

[18] Dagenais M, MacDonald D, Baron M, Hudson M, Tatibouet S, Steele R, et al. The Canadian systemic sclerosis oral health study IV: Oral radiographic manifestations in systemic sclerosis compared with the general population. Oral Surgery, Oral Medicine, Oral Pathology, Oral Radiology. 2015;**120**(2):104-111

[19] Dost F, Farah CS. Stimulating the discussion on saliva substitutes: A clinical perspective. Australian Dental Journal. 2013;**58**:11-17

[20] Tolle SL. Scleroderma: Considerations for dental hygienists. International Journal of Dental Hygiene. 2008;**6**(2):77-83

[21] Farah C, Ashman R, Challacombe S. Oral Candidosis. Clinics in Dermatology. 2000;**18**:553-562

[22] Mays JW, Sarmadi M, Moutsopoulos NM. Oral manifestations of systemic autoimmune and inflammatory diseases: Diagnosis and clinical management. The Journal of Evidence-Based Dental Practice. 2012;**12**(3):265-282

[23] Alantar A, Cabane J, Hachulla E, Princ G, Ginisty D, Hassin M, et al. V recommendations for the care of oral involvement in patients with systemic sclerosis. Arthritis Care and Research. 2011;**63**(8):1126-1133

[24] Wierichs RJ, Meyer-Lueckel H. Systematic review on noninvasive treatment of root caries lesions. Journal of Dental Research. 2015;**94**(2):261-271

[25] Agence Nationale de Sécurité du Médicament et des produits de santé. Prescription des antibiotiques en pratique bucco-dentaire. 2011

[26] Atos Medical. (page consultée le 18/01/2019). Therabite ® Jaw Motion Rehabilitation System™, [en ligne]. https://www.atosmedical. fr/product/therabite-jaw-motion-rehabilitationsystem

[27] Shetty S, Shenoi SD. Autologous platelet-rich fibrin in treatment of scleroderma ulcer. International Wound Journal. 2016;**13**(5):1065

Section 5

# Follicular Occlusion Disorders

Chapter 5

# Hidradenitis Suppurativa

*Salar Hazany, Crystal Zhou, Joshua Bronte, Curtis Tam,*
*Jeffrey Khong and Abhinav Vempati*

## Abstract

Hidradenitis Suppurativa (HS) is a chronic inflammatory skin disorder characterized by painful nodules, abscesses, and tunneled sinus tract formation, predominantly affecting areas rich in apocrine glands. The disease poses significant diagnostic and therapeutic challenges due to its complex pathophysiology and variable clinical presentations. Early detection and intervention are critical in preventing disease progression and minimizing its impact on patients' quality of life. This chapter provides an overview of HS, including diagnostic approaches and management strategies, with a particular focus on surgical interventions. Wide local excision remains the gold standard for achieving long-term remission, but tissue-sparing techniques like deroofing offer effective alternatives, particularly in cases where post-procedural complications or cosmetic concerns are paramount. The role of advanced imaging modalities, such as ultrasound, is also discussed, emphasizing their utility in accurately assessing disease extent and guiding surgical decisions. Through a detailed case study, we highlight the importance of ultrasound guidance in identifying hidden disease processes that may elude conventional clinical evaluation. This chapter aims to provide clinicians with a comprehensive understanding of HS, promoting informed decision-making and improved patient outcomes.

**Keywords:** hidradenitis suppurativa, acne inversa, deroofing, chemical sinusectomy, follicular occlusion

## 1. Introduction

Hidradenitis Suppurativa (HS), also known as acne inversa, is a chronic disease characterized by deep, painful, inflamed nodular lesions, which collect into abscesses connected by complex networks of epithelialized sinus tracts beneath the surface of the skin. Symptoms of HS are painful and can present significant physical and emotional challenges for affected patients. As of 2020, the estimated global prevalence of HS was between 0.0003–4.1% [1]. However, emerging evidence and clinical experience strongly suggest that HS is more widespread than reported in the literature. This section will provide insight on this debilitating, underdiagnosed, and overlooked condition, with clinical insights to guide enhanced treatment selection and administration.

HS flares most commonly affect the axillary, inguinal, perianal, and inframammary regions [1]. These areas are characterized by skin folds that rub against each other constantly, which leads to several concerns. Continual friction and pressure from the performance of repetitive everyday activities not only increases patient discomfort, but progressively exacerbates symptoms over time. These areas are rich in sweat glands, and thus tend to be moist, warm environments facilitating bacterial colonization. Draining abscesses, often accompanied by noticeable odor presenting in these sensitive areas can lead to significant embarrassment and stigmatization, leading to social withdrawal and avoidance of intimacy [2, 3]. Presently, HS lacks both a curative solution and consistent treatment outcomes. Depending on the severity of disease progression, this condition can be debilitating, leading to both physical and psychosocial dysfunction.

Clinical outcomes for HS are closely linked to early disease detection and appropriate management [4]. However, diagnostic delays are significant for this condition, defined by a recent review as between 7.3–10.2 years in adult populations, and 2 years in pediatric patients [4]. Though HS presents cutaneously, patients do not always present to dermatologists for initial symptom resolution, often seeking care at urgent care clinics or emergency rooms for immediate symptom relief [5]. Most patients visit more than 5 physicians before receiving a formal HS diagnosis [5]. In clinical settings where awareness of the condition is low, misdiagnoses are common, as lesions can be mistaken for other pathologies such as sexually transmitted diseases, or lifestyle factors such as weight or lack of hygiene [6]. Repeated misdiagnoses of this nature can be emotionally damaging to patients, contributing to medical fatigue and trauma for an already emotionally vulnerable patient population. In addition, the progression of HS has been linked to squamous cell carcinoma (SCC) development. While reported cases are rare, case reports have documented SCC's potential to develop within preexisting HS lesions (most often those of Hurley Stage III severity) if left untreated [7, 8]. This affinity for evolution into invasive SCC highlights the critical importance of early intervention for this condition [9]. Enhancing understanding of HS will benefit practitioners across various medical specialties, particularly those in primary care, gynecology, oncology, emergency medicine, surgery, and psychiatry, who are likely to encounter this condition.

A variety of factors contribute to HS pathogenesis, including a range of hormonal, genetic, dietary, and mechanical influences [10]. While the biochemical mechanisms remain a subject of research and discordance, HS is clinically understood as a disease of follicular occlusion. Characteristic symptoms of the condition originate from a physical defect that compromises the structural integrity of the pilosebaceous unit in affected individuals. When debris accumulates within these compromised follicles, it becomes trapped and is unable to be expelled to the skin's surface. Instead, the trapped debris and infected material gradually accumulate and worsen over time, creating a positive feedback loop of symptom exacerbation. This leads to the dilation and eventual rupture of the occluded follicular-apocrine unit, causing its contents to leak laterally and subcutaneously. The formation of epithelialized sinus tracts is a consequence of the body's attempt to heal and reconstruct the tubular duct structure of the follicle, although these tracts remain beneath the skin's surface. Sinus tract formation continually compounds inflammatory reactions, creating chronic symptoms that are difficult to manage non-invasively.

## 2. Diagnosis

There is no definitive diagnostic test for HS; diagnosis relies on qualitative clinical assessment. However, once the clinical presentation of HS is understood, its characteristic symptoms provide clear diagnostic criteria.

The Hurley Staging System is widely used to classify HS severity based on morphology, distribution, and chronicity. This system is particularly effective in quickly assessing the severity of HS, especially in Hurley Stage III. It demonstrates moderate inter-rater reliability and substantial inter-rater reliability across all stages [11].

- *Hurley Stage I* is defined as mild HS and is characterized by isolated single or multiple inflammatory nodules without sinus tract formation or scarring.

- *Hurley Stage II* represents moderate HS and is marked by single or multiple recurrent abscesses and nodules with sinus tract formation or scarring, which remain distinctly separated.

- *Hurley Stage III* is the most severe form of HS, presenting with diffuse, multiple recurrent abscesses accompanied by multiple interconnected sinus tracts. These interconnected tracts can be described as "tunneled." This stage of disease progression typically requires surgical intervention for resolution.

Lowered quality of life (QoL) has been well-established among patients with HS [12]. Evaluation of psychosocial metrics with surveys like the Dermatology Life Quality Index (DLQI), or the Hidradenitis Suppurativa Quality of Life (HiSQoL or HSQoL-24) surveys at both initial encounter and routine follow-up is highly encouraged for holistic management of this condition, particularly in cases requiring surgical intervention [13, 14].

## 3. Management

Effective management of hidradenitis suppurativa (HS) begins with early detection and implementation of lifestyle modifications aimed at preventing the formation of new lesions and mitigating the exacerbation of subcutaneous inflammatory processes. Among these, the most significant lifestyle factors include smoking cessation, dietary adjustments, and consciously minimizing pressure and friction in affected areas [4].

A broad spectrum of medical treatments is available for managing the symptoms associated with HS, including oral and topical antibiotics, biologics, hormonal regulation, intralesional corticosteroids, laser, and electrosurgery treatments [1, 4]. Although systemic antibiotics are commonly recommended as a first-line therapy, this approach is largely based on clinician discretion rather than supported by robust scientific evidence. This section will focus primarily on surgical interventions, which currently represent the only curative option for HS.

Treatment selection primarily depends on the severity of disease progression. When considering patients' decisions to initiate treatments for HS, it is critical to understand their priorities and manage expectations realistically, taking into account factors such as pain tolerance, perceptions of treatment risk, treatment fatigue, and overall disease understanding [15].

This section will delve into both established and emerging surgical techniques.

### 3.1 Incision and drainage

Incision and drainage (I&D) is the most commonly reported intervention for HS [16]. This procedure is most appropriate for the relief of acute cases, particularly those characterized by distinct fluctuant nodules and pus accumulation [17]. I&D involves a simple technique, requires minimal specialized equipment, and can be performed quickly in a variety of patient care settings to provide immediate relief from an active HS flare.

Most cases of I&D can be performed under local anesthesia, using topical numbing creams or subcutaneous infiltration. After sterilizing the site and numbing has been achieved, a sharp tool such as a lancet, surgical scissors, or scalpel blade is used to make a single incision through the skin overlying the active HS lesion. Gentle manual pressure is applied adjacent and lateral to the edges of the lesion until total extrusion of abscessed contents is achieved. The wound is then packed, first with a wet dressing such as xeroform gauze to minimize patient discomfort during dressing changes, then with sterile gauze, before being left to heal via secondary intent.

I&D offers only temporary relief of HS symptoms, as it does not remove the underlying diseased tissue that contributes to chronic inflammation and progressive symptom exacerbation. The technique is associated with an almost 100% recurrence rate and should always be coupled with relevant dietary and lifestyle modifications [17]. In most cases, more invasive excisional procedures will be necessary for curative outcomes if symptoms persist or recur. Nonetheless, patients often opt for I&D, fully aware of the risk of recurrence, due to its lower invasiveness and the desire to minimize healing time and scarring [13, 14].

### 3.2 Wide local excision

Wide local excision for HS involves total resection of the implicated tissues until a margin of healthy subcutaneous fat is reached. Many clinicians consider wide local excision the gold standard for HS treatment, as complete resection offers the highest likelihood of successful symptom resolution and the lowest recurrence rates [18]. Wide local excision is often the only option available to resolve symptoms in patients with Hurley stage III HS. However, depending on the extent of disease progression and the anatomical location(s) involved, resecting large quantities of tissue increases the risk of complications during the prolonged healing process and may result in undesirable scar sequelae. Still, most patients report the pain of healing from surgery to be less significant compared to pain during an HS flare, and successful wide local excision has been shown to significantly improve patient QoL [19].

Post operative complications vary depending on the initial severity of disease, individual patient risk factors, and operator-dependent differences in surgical maneuvers. Dehiscence and recurrence are the most commonly reported adverse outcomes, followed by infection, over-granulation, neuroplexia (6%), and hematoma formation (4%) [15, 20]. The choice of wound closure and reconstruction method after surgery remains contentious among practitioners and can determine the risk of post-operative complications [21]. In our clinical practice, secondary intention healing is considered the gold standard due to its lower complication and recurrence rates, as well as a reduced risk of anaerobic bacterial colonization in the wound bed. Despite its advantages in minimizing recurrence, the healing process is typically prolonged and painful, especially in areas subject to high friction, leading to challenging scarring dynamics, including contracture scars that may limit mobility. Primary closure, while expedient, is linked to the highest recurrence rates among closure techniques, associated with a higher likelihood of wound dehiscence and may result in hypertrophic and contracture scars [17, 20].

## 3.3 Deroofing

Surgical deroofing, also known as unroofing, is a tissue-sparing surgical technique that involves the removal of all infected inflammatory tissue overlying HS abscesses, along with the communicating sinus tracts between, but sparing unaffected tissues surrounding them. Using a probe, active abscesses and their associated sinus tracts are carefully identified and thoroughly eradicated. The deroofed wound "floor" is then allowed to heal by secondary intention. This procedure is relatively conservative compared to wide local excision, as it proceeds in an exploratory manner, preserving surrounding unaffected tissue to minimize post-operative complications and undesirable scarring. Although this technique is preferred by patients and associated with lower morbidity rates, it is generally associated with a higher risk of recurrence compared to wide local excision [18]. However, it is also important to note that outcomes with this technique are highly operator-dependent, and studies with robust controls are rare.

In literature, deroofing has been recommended for mild cases of HS (Hurley stage I-II) but the technique is effective even in areas of extensive disease infiltration [16, 17]. The following case study involves a patient with Hurley stage III HS that has persisted for 10 years without medical intervention.

The deroofing procedure took place under local anesthesia, using a ring block with injections of 1% lidocaine with epinephrine combined with bupivacaine in a 1:1 ratio. The patient was positioned in the prone position. A small incision was made in the affected area with a #11 blade. A metal probe was used to identify affected sinuses. Titanium-coated ceramic facelift scissors were used to remove tissue covering affected sinus tracts in the abscess cavity. The cavity was then irrigated with sterile saline solution. The wound was packed with xeroform gauze, covered with sterile dressing, and secured with sterile adhesive strips. The patient tolerated the procedure well with moderate pain and bleeding. The patient was given clear wound care instructions for dressing changes, and appropriate supporting antibiotics and pain management regimen. The patient reports high satisfaction and reports no symptom recurrence at 12 and 24-month follow-up (**Figures 1–3**).

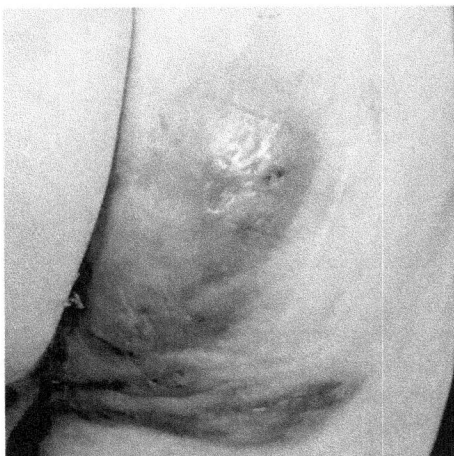

**Figure 1.**
*Pre-Operative photograph of Hurley stage III HS on Fitzpatrick type II skin.*

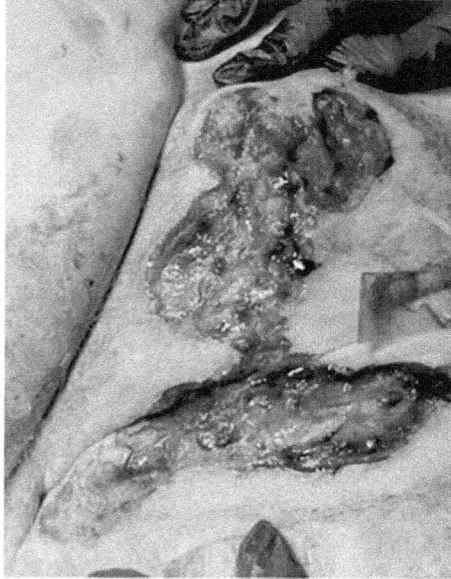

**Figure 2.**
*Post-Operative photograph following surgical deroofing.*

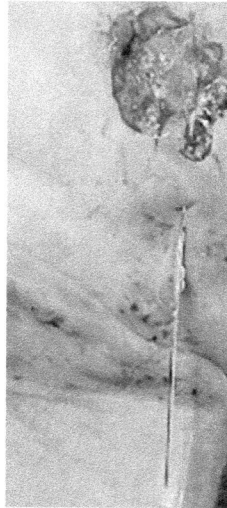

**Figure 3.**
*Lacrimal probe identifying communicating sinus tracts for deroofing.*

Patients often prefer tissue-sparing procedures when available, and deroofing can achieve symptom resolution comparable to wide local excision. The deroofing technique is particularly advantageous for HS cases that carry a high risk of post-procedure complications, functional impairment, or when cosmetic outcomes are a high priority for the patient.

The conservative excision of tissue overlying sinus tracts makes surgical deroofing a largely exploratory procedure, as the full extent of disease progression is often difficult to determine through external physical assessment. Given this uncertainty, patient counseling and informed consent are of paramount importance. It is essential to discuss the lack of a guaranteed outcome, as well as the potential cosmetic and infection risks.

There is significant variability in both the procedure and its outcomes, largely dependent on the operator's skill and the tools used. Additionally, the success of deroofing heavily relies on diligent wound care. Therefore, it is crucial to manage patient expectations, provide detailed aftercare instructions, and ensure regular follow-up visits to monitor healing and address any complications in a timely manner.

## 3.4 Chemical sinusectomy

Chemical sinusectomy is a therapeutic approach that employs strong chemical peeling agents, such as trichloroacetic acid (TCA), to achieve targeted destruction of affected tissues and simultaneous cauterization of proliferative sinus tracts in HS. This method leverages the controlled tissue-destructive properties of TCA, which, upon contact, not only reduces local pro-inflammatory mediators but also creates an acidic environment that may decrease bacterial colonization, a factor contributing to the severity of HS symptoms [22].

TCA is widely used in dermatology to diminish the appearance of aberrant scarring, and by promoting collagen remodeling, it may also contribute to more favorable healing outcomes following its application in HS treatment. The chemical sinusectomy technique represents a minimally invasive alternative to more extensive surgical interventions. Tthe least invasive curative surgical treatment still results in an open wound necessitating significant healing precautions. Chemical sinusectomy overcomes these drawbacks while still specifically targeting the root cause of disease progression.

This approach is particularly advantageous in cosmetically sensitive areas, such as the face, where large-area tissue eradication may be less acceptable. Although chemical sinusectomy is minimally invasive, it typically requires stepwise conservative treatments and carries a higher likelihood of recurrence compared to surgical interventions like deroofing and wide local excision.

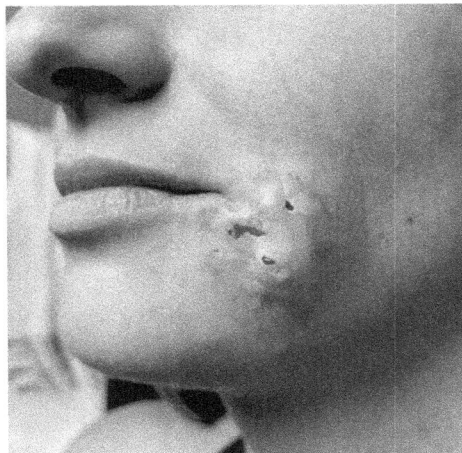

**Figure 4.**
*Post-operative photograph of facial HS on Fitzpatrick type III skin, directly following chemical sinusectomy with 90% TCA.*

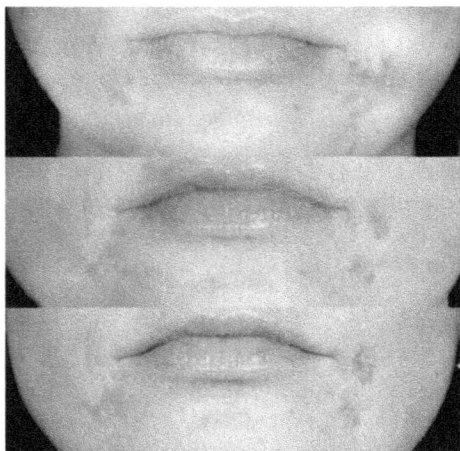

**Figure 5.**
*Photos taken 3–6 weeks apart, between chemical sinusectomy sessions. Note visibly decreased inflammatory activity.*

The following case (**Figures 4** and **5**) shows a patient with HS on the face, which was treated with three rounds of chemical sinusectomy. Local anesthesia was achieved with subcutaneous injections of lidocaine with 1% epinephrine. After the site was sterilized with chlorohexidine, an introducer was used to insert an 18-Gauge blunt-tipped cannula, dipped in 90% TCA solution, into each implicated sinus tract. The patient reported increasing satisfaction with each session of treatment, citing minimal discomfort during the healing process. No recurrence has been reported since 6-month follow up.

## 4. Ultrasound guidance

Ultrasonography serves as an invaluable adjunct in both the diagnostic and management processes for patients with HS [23, 24]. This imaging modality enables clinicians to accurately identify the extent and location of underlying sinus tracts, which is crucial for determining the necessity of surgical intervention. Moreover,

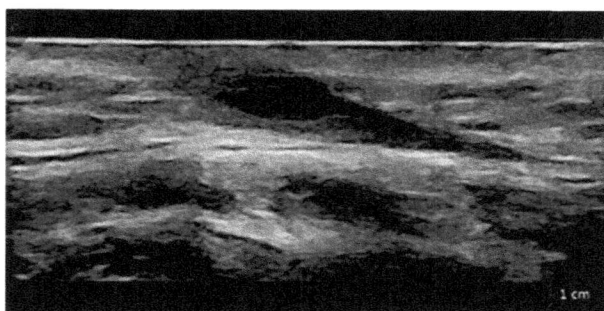

**Figure 6.**
*HS sinus tracts visualized by Clarius L20 HD3 Scanner (8-20 MHz). HS tunnels present as hypoechoic areas relative to surrounding dermal tissues.*

ultrasonography aids in setting realistic patient expectations regarding surgery and postoperative healing, while also guiding precise and targeted tissue removal during surgical procedures [23].

The following case illustrates the critical importance of ultrasound (US) guidance in a case of extensive HS initially misclassified as Hurley Stage II. The patient presented with a single draining lesion in the axilla, causing mild discomfort. Exploratory deroofing was performed under local anesthesia, during which no interconnecting sinuses were identified through probe palpation. Hemostasis was achieved

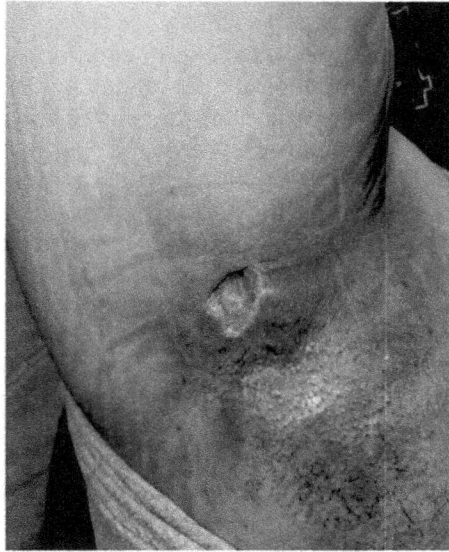

**Figure 7.**
*Post-procedure photograph following minor deroofing of HS lesion.*

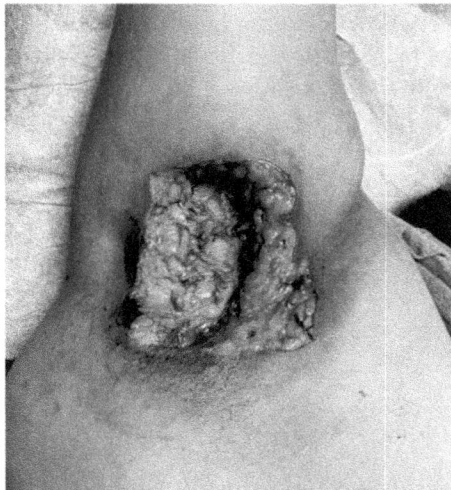

**Figure 8.**
*Post-operative photograph following complete resection of diseased tissues and tunnels.*

using an aluminum chloride solution, and the wound was packed and left to heal by secondary intention.

However, the wound continued to drain over the following days, prompting the patient to return for a follow-up visit. Ultrasound analysis at this visit revealed a deep network of tunnels invading the dermal layers and underlying connective tissue. A second, more extensive procedure was performed, and no recurrence has been reported at the 24-month follow-up (**Figures 6–8**).

## 5. Conclusion

Hidradenitis Suppurativa remains a challenging condition to manage due to its complex pathophysiology, variable clinical presentation, and the significant impact it has on patients' quality of life. The condition's propensity for chronicity and recurrence, coupled with its often debilitating physical and psychosocial effects, underscores the need for comprehensive and individualized treatment strategies.

Early detection and timely intervention are critical in altering the disease course, potentially reducing the severity of symptoms and preventing the progression to more advanced stages. While lifestyle modifications and pharmacological therapies form the foundation of HS management, surgical interventions, particularly tissue-sparing techniques like deroofing, play a pivotal role in achieving long-term symptom resolution. The choice of surgical modality should be guided by the extent of disease progression, anatomical considerations, and patient preferences, with an emphasis on minimizing post-operative complications and preserving function and esthetics.

The importance of advanced diagnostic tools, such as ultrasound, cannot be overstated, as they offer a more accurate assessment of disease severity and guide the extent of surgical intervention. This case study further highlights the role of ultrasound in uncovering hidden disease processes that may not be apparent through physical examination alone.

Ultimately, successful management of HS requires a multidisciplinary approach, involving collaboration across specialties to address the physical, emotional, and psychological needs of patients. As the understanding of HS continues to evolve, ongoing research and clinical experience will undoubtedly refine existing treatment protocols and introduce novel therapeutic options, offering hope for improved outcomes for those affected by this debilitating condition.

*Hidradenitis Suppurativa*
*DOI: http://dx.doi.org/10.5772/intechopen.1007534*

## Author details

Salar Hazany[1*], Crystal Zhou[2], Joshua Bronte[3], Curtis Tam[4], Jeffrey Khong[5] and Abhinav Vempati[4]

1 Scar Healing Institute, Los Angeles, USA

2 UCLA David Geffen School of Medicine, Los Angeles, USA

3 Washington University in St. Louis, Los Angeles, USA

4 Icahn Mount Sinai School of Medicine, New York, USA

5 John Hopkins School of Medicine, Baltimore, USA

*Address all correspondence to: drsalar@hazanyderm.com

IntechOpen

# References

[1] Nguyen TV, Damiani G, Orenstein LAV, Hamzavi I, Jemec GB. Hidradenitis suppurativa: An update on epidemiology, phenotypes, diagnosis, pathogenesis, comorbidities and quality of life. Journal of the European Academy of Dermatology and Venereology. 2021;**35**(1):50-61

[2] Krajewski PK, Strobel A, Schultheis M, Staubach P, Grabbe S, Hennig K, et al. Hidradenitis Suppurativa is associated with severe sexual impairment. Dermatology (Basel, Switzerland). 2024;**240**(2):205-215

[3] Bilgic A, Fettahlıoglu Karaman B, Demirseren DD, Cınar L, Kacar N, Türel Ermertcan A, et al. Internalized stigma in hidradenitis Suppurativa: A Multicenter cross-sectional study. Dermatology (Basel, Switzerland). 2023;**239**(3):445-453

[4] Jenkins T, Isaac J, Edwards A, Okoye GA. Hidradenitis Suppurativa. Dermatologic Clinics. 2023;**41**(3):471-479

[5] Garg A, Neuren E, Cha D, Kirby JS, Ingram JR, Jemec GBE, et al. Evaluating patients' unmet needs in hidradenitis suppurativa: Results from the global survey of impact and healthcare needs (VOICE) project. Journal of the American Academy of Dermatology. 2020;**82**(2):366-376

[6] Nesbitt E, Clements S, Driscoll M. A concise clinician's guide to therapy for hidradenitis suppurativa. International Journal of Women's Dermatology. 2020;**6**(2):80-84

[7] Gierek M, Niemiec P, Szyluk K, Ochala-Gierek G, Bergler-Czop B. Hidradenitis suppurativa and squamous cell carcinoma: A systematic review of the literature. Postepy Dermatologii I Alergologii. 2023;**40**(3):350-354

[8] Atri S, Mahmoud AB, Zehani A, Chammakhi A, Rebai W, Kacem MJ. The management of hidradenitis suppurativa degenerating into squamous cell carcinoma: About three case reports. Annals of Medicine and Surgery. 2021;**64**. Available from: https://journals.lww.com/10.1016/j.amsu.2021.102239 Accessed: 9 September 2024

[9] Juviler PG, Patel AP, Qi Y. Infiltrative squamous cell carcinoma in hidradenitis suppurativa: A case report for early surgical intervention. International Journal of Surgery Case Reports. 2019;**55**:50-53

[10] Alter M. Hidradenitis suppurativa. Dermatology (Heidelberg, Germany). 2024;**75**(6):497-506

[11] Ovadja ZN, Schuit MM, van der Horst CMAM, Lapid O. Inter- and intrarater reliability of Hurley staging for hidradenitis suppurativa. The British Journal of Dermatology. 2019;**181**(2):344-349

[12] Deckers IE, Kimball AB. The handicap of hidradenitis Suppurativa. Dermatologic Clinics. 2016;**34**(1):17-22

[13] Krajewski P, Matusiak Ł, Szepietowska M, Rymaszewska J, Jemec G, Kirby J, et al. Hidradenitis Suppurativa quality of life (HiSQOL): Creation and validation of the polish language version. Advances in Dermatology and Allergology. 2021;**38**(6):967-972

[14] Krajewski PK, Marrón SE, Gomez-Barrera M, Tomas-Aragones L,

Gilaberte-Calzada Y, Szepietowski JC. The use of HSQoL-24 in an assessment of quality-of-life impairment among hidradenitis Suppurativa patients: First look at real-life data. Journal of Clinical Medicine. 2021;**10**(22):5446

[15] Salame N, Sow YN, Siira MR, Garg A, Chen SC, Patzer RE, et al. Factors affecting treatment selection among patients with hidradenitis Suppurativa. JAMA Dermatology. 2024;**160**(2):179-186

[16] Gierek M, Ochała-Gierek G, Kitala D, Łabuś W, Bergler-Czop B. Surgical management of hidradenitis suppurativa. Postepy Dermatologii I Alergologii. 2022;**39**(6):1015-1020

[17] Shukla R, Karagaiah P, Patil A, Farnbach K, Ortega-Loayza AG, Tzellos T, et al. Surgical treatment in hidradenitis Suppurativa. Journal of Clinical Medicine. 2022;**11**(9):2311

[18] Wong HS, Jiang JY, Huang SD, Zhu P, Ji X, Wang DG. A review of surgical and reconstructive techniques for hidradenitis suppurativa. Archives of Dermatological Research. 2024;**316**(6):270

[19] Dick J, Kröhl V, Enk A, Hartschuh W, Gholam P. Improvement in quality of life and pain in patients with hidradenitis Suppurativa after wide local excision: A prospective study. Dermatologic Surgery : Official Publication for American Society for Dermatologic Surgery Al. 2021;**47**(12):1556-1561

[20] Elliott J, Chui K, Rosa N, Reffell L, Jemec B. Hidradenitis suppurativa: A review of post-operative outcomes. The Journal of Plastic, Reconstructive and Aesthetic Surgery. 2021;**74**(3):644-710

[21] Tang B, Huang Z, Yi Q, Zheng X. Complications of hidradenitis suppurativa after surgical management: A systematic review and meta-analysis. International Wound Journal. 2023;**20**(4):1253-1261

[22] Kim MS, Lim JH, Jin YJ, Jang JH, Hah JH. Trichloroacetic acid Chemocauterization: A simple method to close small Tracheocutaneous fistula. The Annals of Otology, Rhinology, and Laryngology. 2016;**125**(8):644-647

[23] Mendes-Bastos P, Martorell A, Bettoli V, Matos AP, Muscianisi E, Wortsman X. The use of ultrasound and magnetic resonance imaging in the management of hidradenitis suppurativa: A narrative review. The British Journal of Dermatology. 2023;**188**(5):591-600

[24] Wortsman X, Calderon P, Castro A. Seventy-MHz ultrasound detection of early signs linked to the severity, patterns of keratin fragmentation, and mechanisms of generation of collections and tunnels in hidradenitis Suppurativa. Journal of Ultrasound in Medicine. 2020;**39**(5):845-857

Chapter 6

# Surgical Management of Hidradenitis Suppurativa

*Lennart Ocker, Nessr Abu Rached and Falk G. Bechara*

## Abstract

The treatment of Hidradenitis suppurativa (HS) is complex and based on different treatment pillars, that often have to be combined in an individual and patient-oriented approach. Surgery is mainly reserved for advanced diseases with irreversible tissue remodeling, such as fistulas, contractions, and scarring. Moreover, surgical treatment may also be considered to achieve drainage and rapid pain relief in acute inflammatory lesions, however, relapse rates are high in these cases and often definitive surgery is required in the course of the disease. This chapter focuses on surgery as an integral component of HS treatment and provides an overview of different surgical techniques. Furthermore, recommendations for the surgical approach to HS patients and perioperative management are also discussed.

**Keywords:** surgery, hidradenitis suppurativa, chronic inflammation, multimodal therapy, imaging, surgical techniques, wound management

## 1. Introduction

Historically, Hidradenitis suppurativa (HS) was considered to be a primarily sweat gland-based disease with radical surgical resection of sweat gland-bearing areas being the only curative treatment [1]. The widely used Pollock procedure allowed a simultaneous bilateral surgical resection of the axillary area followed by primary wound closure [2, 3]. In 1989, Hurley described a classification system, which allows an effective differentiation of HS patients from a surgical point of view and is still continuously used in clinical practice [4].

HS is currently understood as a chronic inflammatory skin disease, affecting primarily the intertriginous, apocrine gland-bearing areas, characterized by recurring inflammatory skin lesions, such as nodules and abscesses. In advanced stages of the disease, chronic inflammation promotes progredient and irreversible tissue destruction through fibrosis, tissue remodeling, and scarring [5]. In this understanding of the disease, early initiation of anti-inflammatory systemic therapy is of great importance to ideally prevent irreversible tissue damage [6]. With a better understanding of HS pathophysiology and the development of effective targeted anti-inflammatory medical therapies, the therapeutic spectrum of HS has evolved [7]. In this context, the surgical approach to HS has shifted from radical prophylactic surgical interventions to a more targeted and, if possible, minimal-invasive approach, leaving healthy and unaffected tissue in place [8]. In the modern therapeutic spectrum of HS,

IntechOpen

surgery represents a fundamental pillar and should be combined with medical anti-inflammatory treatments and supportive non-medical therapies in a multimodal and patient-oriented approach [7].

Indications for surgery are versatile and include acute inflammatory disease as well as the treatment of chronic irreversible tissue damage [9]. In this chapter, the authors describe established surgical techniques and comprehensive surgical treatment approaches for HS.

## 2. Perioperative considerations

Surgery in HS can be performed in an out-patient or in-patient treatment setting, depending on the extent of surgery, patient characteristics, and patient's preference. Preoperative communication with the patient should establish a clear treatment plan including postoperative wound care, physiotherapy, and pain management. Potential surgical risks should be addressed and patients should also be informed about the possibility of an intraoperative variation of resection margins, as clinical evaluation of lesions is often more specific intraoperatively compared to the preoperative setting. Patient should become empowered to be actively involved in their own recovery and rehabilitation, which results in increased levels of autonomy and control post-surgery and improved treatment outcomes [10].

In general, clinical assessment of surgical margins is sufficient for HS surgery. However, in cases of advanced disease or high inflammatory activity, demarcation lines of HS lesions may be blurred. Preoperative imaging can provide an improved evaluation of surgical margins, particularly in complex areas or where infiltration of anatomical structures is suspected [11].

Ultrasonography (US) represents an established and widely used imaging tool in dermatologic surgery. Sonographic features of HS include a thickened, hypoechogenic dermis, pseudocystic lesions, anechoic fluid collections, increased peripheral vascularization, and hypoechoic interconnected fistulous tracts (**Figure 1**) [12]. In HS, the US can contribute to an enhanced visualization of the surgical area, allowing a more targeted surgical approach and reducing the risk of postoperative recurrence [13].

Magnetic resonance imaging (MRI) in HS mainly uses sequences with T2-weighted acquisitions and short tau inversion recovery (STIR) to enhance the

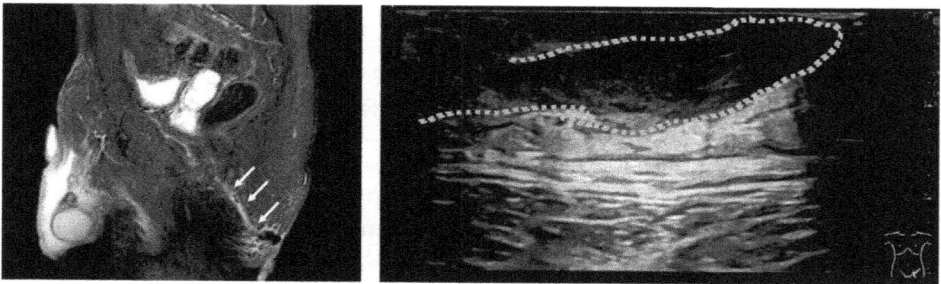

**Figure 1.**
*Visualization of a pararectal infralevatory fistula in magnetic resonance imaging (MRI), T2-sequence, sagittal view (left). Sonographic image of a deep-reaching subcutaneous fistula in the left groin area, clinical margins marked with orange dots (right). (pictures courtesy Department of Dermatologic Surgery, Ruhr-university Bochum).*

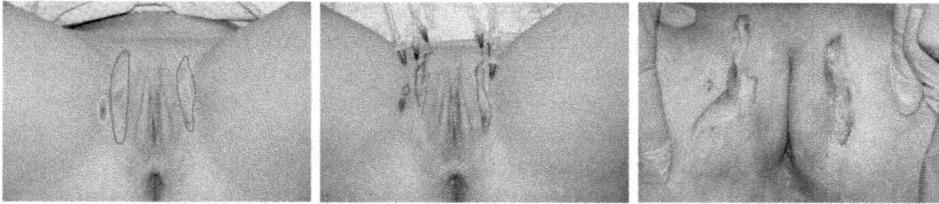

**Figure 2.**
*Left: Preoperative situs with marked lesions (red: Fistula, green: Nodule); middle: Tumescence local anesthesia. Surgical margins are marked preoperatively; right: Completed surgical excision of the bilateral fistulas and deroofing of a nodule under tumescence local anesthesia. (pictures courtesy Department of Dermatologic Surgery, Ruhr-university Bochum).*

signal of fluid collections [14]. Especially in the perineal and perianal region, MRI can improve the demarcation of HS lesions and can facilitate a differentiation from Crohn's disease (**Figure 1**) [11].

Ideally, surgery in HS should be performed in periods of low inflammatory activity to facilitate clinical demarcation of lesions and reliable determination of surgical margins. In cases with highly inflammatory surgical sites and extensive drainage, pre- or perioperative anti-inflammatory therapies are often engaged to optimize surgical conditions. Perioperative combinations with anti-inflammatory therapies, including systemic antibiotics or targeted therapies, have been shown to improve treatment outcomes and reduce the risk of recurrence [15–17].

Another important aspect of HS surgery represents the selection of sufficient perioperative anesthesia and postoperative pain management [18]. While localized surgical resections can be performed under local anesthesia, extensive surgery may require general anesthesia. Tumescent local anesthesia (TLA), a subtype of local anesthesia, uses diluted local anesthetic solutions that are injected into the surgical area to achieve tissue hydro-dissection and improve surgical conditions (**Figure 2**) [19]. In HS surgery, TLA is widely used for extensive surgical areas and may be combined with other anesthesiology methods, such as general anesthesia. TLA has been reported to improve surgical conditions through tissue hydro-dissection, reduced intraoperative bleeding, and reduced postoperative pain [19]. Also, a sufficient postoperative analgetic regimen should be established in the preoperative setting and may be adapted in the postoperative course following current guidelines [20].

## 3. Surgical techniques

Various surgical treatment approaches and techniques have been described for HS in the literature. However, surgical therapy is often performed in an individualized approach and inconsistent nomenclature was a major concern in the past. To enable higher standardization and comparability of surgical techniques in HS surgery, standardized definitions were developed in a Delphi consensus statement further specifying excisional and deroofing procedures depending on their site and extent [21].

### 3.1 Incision and drainage

Incision and drainage (I&D) is defined as "incision of skin with the intent to drain a collection of fluid" and represents a widely used and easy-to-perform surgical procedure for the treatment of skin and soft tissue abscesses [21, 22]. As the effect of local anesthesia is limited in acute inflammatory tissue, this procedure is often performed under cryo-anesthesia and/or sedation. After drainage is established, the wound cavity should be copiously irrigated with sterile normal saline solution. Tamponade is only recommended for abscesses greater than 5 cm in diameter and has not been shown to reduce recurrence rates [23].

Taking into account the chronic course of HS, incisions are associated with a high relapse rate and therefore cannot be considered a definitive treatment [24]. Nevertheless, incision and drainage may be implemented in a multimodal treatment concept as an exit strategy for highly inflammatory cases, when rapid symptom relief is desired. As deroofing can be performed in approximately the same amount of time, guidelines recommend deroofing over incision and drainage [7].

## 3.2 Deroofing

Deroofing describes a minimally invasive surgical procedure to remove the top layer ("the roof") of inflammatory nodules, abscesses, solitary fistulas, or scars, leading to the exposure of its ground [25]. Incisions are usually performed in a diagonal cutting shape and followed by curettage of gelatinous mass and secondary intention healing (**Figure 3**). The advantages over excisional procedures are the simplicity of the procedure, low complication rates, reduced wound healing time, and high patient satisfaction [26]. Moreover, deroofing can be combined with other techniques in an individualized surgical approach if required [27].

Effective deroofing procedures have also been reported using $CO_2$-laser ablation followed by secondary intention healing. This variant was associated with a faster time to wound re-epithelialization [28, 29].

"Skin-tissue-sparing excision with electrosurgical peeling" (STEEP) represents a similar electrosurgical treatment approach with successive tangential excisions, that are performed with an electrosurgical wire loop until the epithelialized bottom of the lesion is exposed, while saving as much healthy tissue as possible [30]. Although this surgical technique is associated with a short time for wound healing and a low risk of wound contraction, no long-term outcomes are reported and evidence is limited to small case series [31].

## 3.3 Excisions

The surgical procedure of excision in HS describes the complete resection of the irreversible tissue damage into healthy, non-affected subcutaneous tissue and is

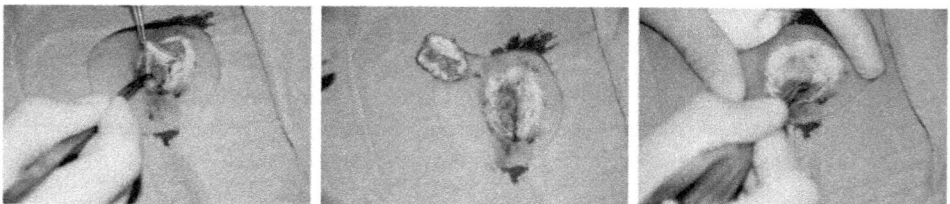

**Figure 3.**
*Deroofing of a subcutaneous abscess. Tangential resection of the lesion's roof (left), uncovering the ground of the lesion with gelatinous granulation tissue (middle), and subsequent curettage of the granulation tissue followed by secondary intention healing (right). (pictures courtesy Department of Dermatologic Surgery, Ruhr-university Bochum).*

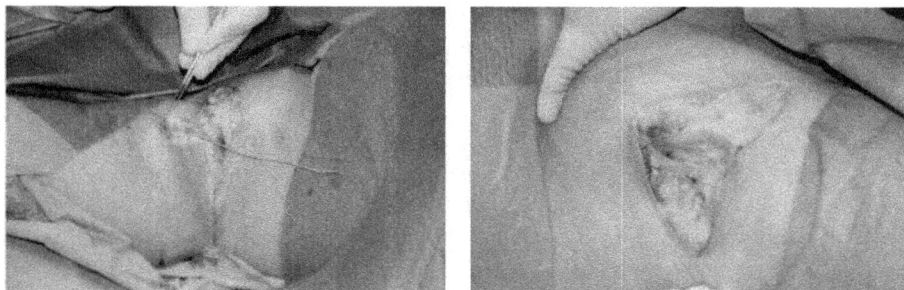

**Figure 4.**
*Excision of a fistula in the right axilla. Intraoperative visualization of the fistula using a surgical probe (left).*
*A surgical defect is left to secondary intention healing (right). (pictures courtesy Department of Dermatologic*
*Surgery, Ruhr-university Bochum).*

considered as first-line treatment option in HS surgery [21]. Based on the extent of the procedure, some authors differentiate between limited or localized, wide, and radical excisions [18]. Following the recent consensus statement on surgical proce-dures in HS, excisions should be categorized depending on the procedural location in lesional or regional excisions and their extent in partial and complete excisions [21]. With the development and implementation of effective anti-inflammatory systemic treatments, the concept of HS surgery has shifted away from extensive resections including non-affected tissue as a "safety margin" to more targeted approaches.

In this procedure, the cutis around the preoperatively marked lesions is cut, fol-lowed by a careful preparation of the lesion along the demarcation lines. Fistulas can be visualized intraoperatively using a probe or medical dyes such as methylene-blue, enabling a targeted surgical resection of the marked lesions (**Figure 4**). To prevent unnecessary deep preparation, the authors recommend a step-wise approach gripping the tissue with surgical clamps and applying light tension to facilitate preparation and tissue dissection. During surgery, fibrotic bands and scar contractures should also be dissolved to prevent postoperative wound contraction and movement restrictions. If possible, as much healthy and unaffected tissue should be left in place to improve postoperative wound healing.

## 4. Wound closure options

A variety of surgical approaches to wound closure have been described for HS includ-ing secondary intention healing, primary wound closure, skin grafting, and skin flaps. As there is no general consensus on the best option, the selection of wound closure is individual and depends on different factors such as the extent and location of the surgi-cal area, disease-specific factors, patient compliance, and the surgeon's preference and experience [32]. More importantly, an adequate and complete resection of the involved irreversibly destructed tissue is crucial before considering wound closure.

In the recent literature, varying recurrence rates have been found for different wound closure options in HS patients with the lowest recurrence rates after secondary intention healing or skin grafting and the highest rates after the use of skin flaps and primary wound closure [33–35].

In HS, secondary intention healing is an established alternative to direct wound closure approaches and describes the successive closure of a postoperative wound through all stages of the physiological wound healing process (**Figure 5**) [36]. Secondary intention healing allows a direct postoperative mobilization and enables early reintegration into the patient's daily life [37]. In contrast to other wound closure options, there is no risk of flap or graft loss. Potential disadvantages include a prolonged time to complete wound healing with often need for specialized wound management and painful wound dressings. Physiotherapeutic support and scar massage are crucial to reduce the risk of postoperative wound contractions and prevent movement restrictions through fibrosis and scarring [37]. In most postoperative HS defects, secondary intention healing can be considered as a first-line wound closure option providing excellent long-term outcomes and a low risk of recurrence [33, 38].

Skin grafting is another wound closure option for extensive surgical defects. Most commonly, split-thickness skin grafts (STSG) are used in HS, as they allow coverage of all anatomic regions with the perineal, gluteal, genital, and inguinal areas being the most frequent application sites. Skin grafting can either be performed immediately after surgical excision of involved areas or in a staged approach after sufficient wound granulation is established, often leading to favorable postoperative outcomes. In clinical trials, STSG has been shown to reduce the time to wound healing in comparison to secondary intention healing and was associated with a reduced risk of wound contraction [39]. Another advantage of skin grafts is the coverage of large surgical defects. If needed, the use of meshed skin grafts can even provide larger defect coverage [40]. Possible limitations of skin grafting include the need for post-coverage patient immobilization to ensure graft healing, adequate postoperative wound management with moisture control, and donor site complications [37]. After graft take is established, the initiation of physiotherapy and scar massage is essential to ensure an optimal postoperative outcome (**Figure 6**).

Negative pressure wound therapy (NPWT) represents an adjunctive option for complex surgical wounds and improves the wound healing process through increasing wound oxygenation and reducing the bacterial wound load [41]. In HS, NPWT can be implemented for the postoperative treatment after extensive surgical resections and may be followed by either secondary intention healing or skin grafting [42].

Primary wound closure describes the adaption of surgical excision margins and may be considered after limited resections. The advantages of this relatively easy-to-perform approach are improved wound healing through definitive closure and

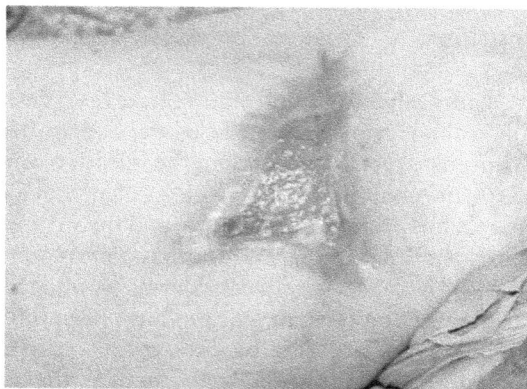

**Figure 5.**
*Secondary intention wound healing four weeks after excision in the axilla region. (pictures courtesy Department of Dermatologic Surgery, Ruhr-university Bochum).*

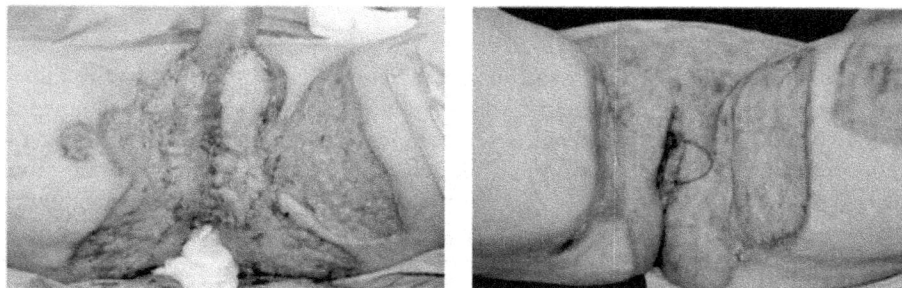

**Figure 6.**
*Split-thickness skin grafting of the genital-perianal area after extensive surgical excisions. Postoperative view after STSG-coverage of scrotum and perineum in a male patient (left). Postoperative result six months after radical excision of the genitofemoral region followed by meshed STSG coverage. Blue loops indicate intraoperatively marked vaginal fistulas (right). (pictures courtesy Department of Dermatologic Surgery, Ruhr-university Bochum).*

favorable esthetic outcomes [43]. However, primary wound closure is primarily limited through defect size and has shown to be associated with a high risk of recurrence (up to 15%) and a risk of postoperative wound dehiscence and surgical site infection [33].

Flaps are another advanced surgical option for postoperative definitive wound closure in HS. A variety of flaps have been described for the reconstruction/coverage of surgical defects of the axilla including transposition flaps, advancement flaps, myocutaneous flaps (**Figure 7**), and fascio-cutaneous flaps, respectively [44–48]. Skin flaps provide accelerated wound healing, enabling early postoperative patient mobilization, and are associated with a reduced risk of postoperative contractions due to scarring [37]. However, studies have reported higher recurrence rates of up to 8% and recent guidelines do not consider skin flaps as a first-line option for wound closure in HS [33]. In specific cases, especially when critical anatomical structures like nerves, vascular structures, or musculature are exposed, the use of skin flaps may be necessary [49].

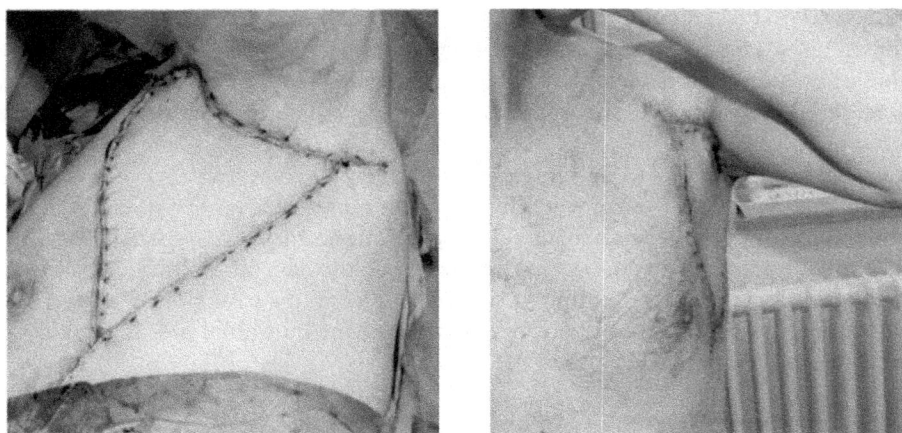

**Figure 7.**
*Surgical reconstruction after resection of the axilla region with a VY-myocutaneous island flap. Left: Intraoperative view after wound closure. Right: Postoperative result after 6 weeks with improved mobility of the shoulder. (pictures courtesy Department of Dermatologic Surgery, Ruhr-university Bochum).*

## 5. Postoperative wound management

In HS, postoperative wound management marks an essential factor in the successful surgical treatment of patients. Depending on the type and extent of surgical procedure, modality of wound closure, wound localization, and patient-specific factors, wound care in HS can be complex. The selection of sufficient wound dressings for the particular wound healing phase is crucial to maintain a moist and clean wound microenvironment [50]. Postoperative physiotherapy, patient mobilization, and scar massage are necessary to achieve optimal functional outcomes [37].

To ensure a seamless transition from operation to post-surgical care, wound management should already be coordinated in the preoperative phase. Depending on the complexity and location of the wound and patient characteristics, wound dressings can either be performed by the patient or family members or by a specialized outpatient nursing service. To optimize postoperative outcomes, patients should become self-empowered by involving them in wound care through information and basic training [51]. Regular postoperative follow-ups should be scheduled to control wound healing and adjust wound care if needed.

## 6. Postoperative complications and surgical challenges in HS

Postoperative complications can be divided into short-term and long-term complications depending on their time of occurrence. Short-term postoperative complications include postoperative bleeding, pain, and surgical site infections. Long-term postoperative complications include wound healing disorders, local recurrence, and contractures associated with scarring.

### 6.1 Short-term complications

Postoperative bleeding typically occurs within the few days after surgery and is often associated with the fading effect of tumescence local anesthesia, intake of anticoagulants, or coagulation disorders. Extensive or prolonged bleeding can lead to decreased levels of hemoglobin and may require transfusion. To prevent postoperative bleeding, meticulous intraoperative hemostasis with electrocoagulation and ligation of small vessels is recommended. Moreover, intraoperative drainage inlay can be considered in wounds with primary closure or flap coverage to prevent hematoma formation.

Surgical site infections (SSI) represent a relatively rare complication in HS surgery. In a retrospective study, the highest SSI rates were reported after incision and drainage procedures, which were performed in obese patients or in an outpatient setting [52]. Clinical warning signs indicating SSI are worsening pain, swelling, increased drainage, and localized overheating of the wound. Wound swaps should be extracted to allow microbiological identification and targeted antimicrobial therapy, taking into account microbiological resistance [53].

### 6.2 Long-term complications

Recurrence within the surgical site marks a major postoperative complication with varying incidence rates reported in the literature. However, there is no standardized definition of recurrence, making comparative analyses difficult. The risk of recurrence depends on various factors, such as resection technique, wound closure modality, the surgeon's expertise, and patient-specific factors [18, 33, 34, 54]. In the concept of HS as a chronic inflammatory disorder, surgery has often to be combined with systemic anti-inflammatory therapy to achieve disease control and prevent recurrence [7]. Prospective clinical studies are needed to examine the effect of multi-modal medical and surgical combination therapies [15].

Postoperative wound contractures can occur as a result of extensive scarring. Large excisions in the axillary region with secondary intention healing are at increased risk for the development of scar contractures, which can result in impaired mobility of the shoulder [18]. Postoperative mobilization of the patient with physiotherapeutic support and stretching of the wounds are crucial factors in wound management to prevent contractures and mobility impairment [37].

## 6.3 Surgical challenges in HS surgery

Chronic inflammatory HS of the perineal and perianal area with advanced irreversible tissue destruction represents a particular challenge for surgery as lesions can extend to critical anatomical structures, such as the rectum, sphincter muscu-lature, or vagina. In these cases, the authors recommend a staged approach with the preoperative establishment of a non-inflammatory surgical field to enable optimal clinical evaluation of the disease. In suspected cases, further imaging (sonography or MRI) and endoscopic diagnostics can be considered [11]. Intraoperatively, cautious preparation of fistulas in the perianal area is recommended with the greatest possible protection of the sphincter musculature. The authors recommend an intraoperative proctological examination in case of extensive perianal fistulas [55]. When anal fistulas are present, temporally inlays of seton or loop drainage can be performed till definitive surgical therapy. Another specific complication, mainly after previous insufficient surgeries, is blind ending tracts and/or cavities that can extend deep parallel to the rectum. Lay-opening of these structures under preservation of the sphincter muscle can be challenging [55]. Consequently, in patients with extensive perianal HS, an individual decision toward an interdisciplinary approach including colorectal surgery should be discussed.

Moreover, the gluteal and perianal areas represent risk zones for the development of cutaneous squamous cell carcinoma, a rare but often fatal complication of long-standing inflammatory HS [56]. These tumors may present as unspecific ulcerations or indurated nodules and can mimic draining openings of sinus tracts or disturbed wound healing. To enable diagnosis in early tumor stages, biopsies of clinically atypi-cal lesions should be performed on a low threshold and referred to histopathologic examination [56]. In locally limited disease, complete tumor resection with wide security margins can be curative. However, most of these tumors are diagnosed in an advanced stage with locoregional or distant metastasis and are then associated with a poor prognosis and high mortality. In these cases, systemic tumor therapies, radio-therapy, and palliative care may be considered as possible treatment options [57].

Recurrence of lesions within the surgical field represents a common complica-tion of HS and may be a result of inadequate previous surgery, insufficient disease control, and patient characteristics [34, 54, 58]. Often, the demarcation of HS lesions is blurred within scarring of previous surgical interventions, making surgical treat-ment of these patients challenging. The authors recommend a step-wise approach, starting with establishing disease control and reducing inflammatory activity prior to re-surgery [7, 16]. In some cases, preoperative imaging can facilitate the adequate evaluation of the extent of lesions; however, precise intraoperative inspection and radical resection of the affected tissue are crucial to prevent further recurrence and establish disease control.

Post-inflammatory lymphedema is a relatively rare but debilitating complication of long-standing severe HS and most commonly affects the scrotum, penis, perineum, and labia majora [59, 60]. Chronic inflammation marks a major risk factor for impairment of lymphatic drainage and the development of secondary lymphedema [61]. Genital lymphedema can cause serious esthetic and functional impairment, and sexual dysfunction and may worsen the quality of life in affected patients [62]. Lymphedema in HS is often accompanied by severe and complex fistulas in the tissue. These patients often require professional interdisciplinary care including conservative and surgical treatment strategies to improve disease control and sexual function [59]. Complete decongestive therapy (CDT) with manual lymphatic drainage and medical anti-inflammatory therapy are established conservative approaches [63, 64]. The recommendations for surgical treatment of these patients are limited to case reports and include the radical resection of affected skin followed by coverage of the genital area with skin grafts [60, 65, 66].

## Conflict of interest

L.O. has received honoraria as a speaker from Novartis Pharma GmbH. F.G.B. has received honoraria for participation in advisory boards, in clinical trials, and/or as a speaker from AbbVie Inc., AbbVie Deutschland GmbH & Co. KG, Boehringer Ingelheim Pharma GmbH & Co. KG, Novartis Pharma GmbH, UCB Pharma, Incyte Corporation, JanssenCilag GmbH, and MoonLake. The funders had no role in the design of the publication, analyses, or interpretation of data; in the writing of the manuscript; or in the decision to publish the results. N.A.R. declares no conflict of interest.

## Author details

Lennart Ocker*, Nessr Abu Rached and Falk G. Bechara
Department of Dermatology, Venereology and Allergology, International Centre for Hidradenitis Suppurativa/Acne Inversa (ICH), Ruhr-University Bochum, Bochum, Germany

*Address all correspondence to: lennart.ocker@kklbo.de

## IntechOpen

# References

[1] Robertshaw D. Surgical treatment of hyperhidrosis and chronic hidradenitis suppurativa. The Journal of Investigative Dermatology. 1974;**63**(1):174-182

[2] Tasche C, Angelats J, Jayaram B. Surgical treatment of hidradenitis suppurativa of the axilla. Plastic and Reconstructive Surgery. 1975;**55**(5):559-562

[3] Pollock WJ, Virnelli FR, Ryan RF. Axillary hidradenitis suppurativa. A simple and effective surgical technique. Plastic and Reconstructive Surgery. 1972;**49**(1):22-27

[4] Hurley HJ. Axillary hyperhidrosis, apocrine bromhidrosis, hidradenitis suppurativa and familial benign pemphigus: Surgical approach. In: Roenigk & Roenigk's Dermatologic Surgery: Principles and Practice. 2nd ed.2 ed. New York: Marcel Dekker Inc.; 1996. pp. 623-646

[5] Sabat R, Jemec GBE, Matusiak Ł, Kimball AB, Prens E, Wolk K. Hidradenitis suppurativa. Nature Reviews Disease Primers. 2020;**6**(1):1-20

[6] Marzano AV, Genovese G, Casazza G, Moltrasio C, Dapavo P, G M. Evidence for a 'window of opportunity' in hidradenitis suppurativa treated with adalimumab: A retrospective, real-life multicentre cohort study*. The British Journal of Dermatology. 2021;**184**(1):133-140

[7] Ocker L, Abu Rached N, Seifert C, Scheel C, Bechara FG. Current medical and surgical treatment of hidradenitis Suppurativa-a comprehensive review. Journal of Clinical Medicine. 2022;**11**(23):7240

[8] Goldberg SR, George R, Bechara FG. 23 - operative techniques for hidradenitis Suppurativa. In: Shi VY, Hsiao JL, Lowes MA, Hamzavi IH, editors. A Comprehensive Guide to Hidradenitis Suppurativa [Internet]. Philadelphia: Elsevier; 2022. pp. 226-232. Verfügbar unter: https://www.sciencedirect.com/science/article/pii/B9780323777247000231 [zitiert: Februar 19, 2024]

[9] Alikhan A, Sayed C, Alavi A, Alhusayen R, Brassard A, Burkhart C. North American clinical management guidelines for hidradenitis suppurativa: A publication from the United States and Canadian hidradenitis Suppurativa foundations: Part I: Diagnosis, evaluation, and the use of complementary and procedural management. Journal of the American Academy of Dermatology. 2019;**81**(1):76-90

[10] Schmidt M, Eckardt R, Scholtz K, Neuner B, von Dossow-Hanfstingl V, Sehouli J. Patient empowerment improved perioperative quality of care in cancer patients aged ≥ 65 years – A randomized controlled trial. PLoS One. 2015;**10**(9):e0137824

[11] Mendes-Bastos P, Martorell A, Bettoli V, Matos AP, Muscianisi E, Wortsman X. The use of ultrasound and magnetic resonance imaging in the management of hidradenitis suppurativa: A narrative review. The British Journal of Dermatology. 2023;**188**(5):591-600

[12] Crisan D, Wortsman X, Alfageme F, Catalano O, Badea A, Scharffetter-Kochanek K. Ultrasonography in dermatologic surgery: Revealing the unseen for improved surgical planning. JDDG Journal der Deutschen Dermatologischen Gesellschaft. 2022;**20**(7):913-926

[13] Cuenca-Barrales C, Salvador-Rodríguez L, Arias-Santiago S, Molina-Leyva A. Pre-operative ultrasound planning in the surgical management of patients with hidradenitis suppurativa. Journal of the European Academy of Dermatology and Venereology. 2020;**34**(10):2362-2367

[14] Srisajjakul S, Prapaisilp P, Bangchokdee S. Magnetic resonance imaging of hidradenitis suppurativa: A focus on the anoperineal location. Korean Journal of Radiology. 2022;**23**(8):785-793

[15] Bechara FG, Podda M, Prens EP, Horváth B, Giamarellos-Bourboulis EJ, Alavi A. Efficacy and safety of adalimumab in conjunction with surgery in moderate to severe hidradenitis suppurativa: The SHARPS randomized clinical trial. JAMA Surgery. 2021;**156**(11):1001-1009

[16] DeFazio MV, Economides JM, King KS, Han KD, Shanmugam VK, Attinger CE. Outcomes after combined radical resection and targeted biologic therapy for the management of recalcitrant hidradenitis suppurativa. Annals of Plastic Surgery. 2016;**77**(2):217

[17] Shanmugam VK, Mulani S, McNish S, Harris S, Buescher T, Amdur R. Longitudinal observational study of hidradenitis suppurativa: Impact of surgical intervention with adjunctive biologic therapy. International Journal of Dermatology. 2018;**57**(1):62-69

[18] Shukla R, Karagaiah P, Patil A, Farnbach K, Ortega-Loayza AG, Tzellos T. Surgical treatment in hidradenitis suppurativa. Journal of Clinical Medicine. 2022;**11**(9):2311

[19] Uttamani RR, Venkataram A, Venkataram J, Mysore V. Tumescent anesthesia for dermatosurgical procedures other than liposuction. Journal of Cutaneous and Aesthetic Surgery. 2020;**13**(4):275-282

[20] Horn R, Kramer J. Postoperative Pain Control. Treasure Island (FL): StatPearls Publishing; 2024. Verfügbar unter: http://www.ncbi.nlm.nih.gov/books/NBK544298/ [zitiert: Februar 9, 2024]

[21] Bui H, Bechara FG, George R, Goldberg S, Hamzavi I, Kirby JS. Surgical procedural definitions for hidradenitis suppurativa developed by expert delphi consensus. JAMA Dermatology. 2023;**159**(4):441-447

[22] Pastorino A, Tavarez MM. Incision and Drainage. Treasure Island (FL): StatPearls Publishing; 2024. Verfügbar unter: http://www.ncbi.nlm.nih.gov/books/NBK556072/ [zitiert: Februar 8, 2024]

[23] Kessler DO, Krantz A, Mojica M. Randomized trial comparing wound packing to no wound packing following incision and drainage of superficial skin abscesses in the pediatric emergency department. Pediatric Emergency Care. 2012;**28**(6):514-517

[24] Zouboulis C, Desai N, Emtestam L, Hunger R, Ioannides D, Juhász I. European S1 guideline for the treatment of hidradenitis suppurativa/acne inversa. Journal of the European Academy of Dermatology and Venereology. 2015;**29**(4):619-644

[25] van der Zee HH, Prens EP, Boer J. Deroofing: A tissue-saving surgical technique for the treatment of mild to moderate hidradenitis suppurativa lesions. Journal of the American Academy of Dermatology. 2010;**63**(3):475-480

[26] Krajewski PK, Sanz-Motilva V, Flores Martinez S, Solera M, Ochando G, Jfri A. Deroofing: A safe, effective and

well-tolerated procedure in patients with hidradenitis suppurativa. Journal of the European Academy of Dermatology and Venereology JEADV. 2024;**38**(5):931-936

[27] Dahmen RA, Gkalpakiotis S, Mardesicova L, Arenberger P, Arenbergerova M. Deroofing followed by thorough sinus tract excision: A modified surgical approach for hidradenitis suppurativa. Journal der Deutschen Dermatologischen Gesellschaft. 2019;**17**(7):698-702

[28] Finley EM, Ratz JL. Treatment of hidradenitis suppurativa with carbon dioxide laser excision and second-intention healing. Journal of the American Academy of Dermatology. 1996;**34**(3):465-469

[29] Hazen PG, Hazen BP. Hidradenitis suppurativa: Successful treatment using carbon dioxide laser excision and marsupialization. Dermatologic Surgery. 2010;**36**(2):208-213

[30] Blok JL, Spoo JR, Leeman FWJ, Jonkman MF, Horváth B. Skin-tissue-sparing excision with electrosurgical peeling (STEEP): A surgical treatment option for severe hidradenitis suppurativa Hurley stage II/III. Journal of the European Academy of Dermatology and Venereology JEADV. 2015;**29**(2):379-382

[31] Janse IC, Hellinga J, Blok JL, van den Heuvel ER, Spoo JR, Jonkman MF. Skin-tissue-sparing excision with electrosurgical peeling: A case series in hidradenitis suppurativa. Acta Dermato-Venereologica. 2016;**96**(3):390-391

[32] Scholl L, Hessam S, Reitenbach S, Bechara FG. Operative behandlungsoptionen bei hidradenitis suppurativa/acne inversa. Der Hautarzt. 2018;**69**(2):149-161

[33] Mehdizadeh A, Hazen PG, Bechara FG, Zwingerman N, Moazenzadeh M, Bashash M. Recurrence of hidradenitis suppurativa after surgical management: A systematic review and meta-analysis. Journal of the American Academy of Dermatology. 2015;**73**(5 Suppl. 1):S70-S77

[34] Ovadja ZN, Zugaj M, Jacobs W, van der Horst CMAM, Lapid O. Recurrence rates following reconstruction strategies after wide excision of hidradenitis suppurativa: A systematic review and meta-analysis. Dermatologic Surgery. 2021;**47**(4):e106-e110

[35] Rompel R, Petres J. Long-term results of wide surgical excision in 106 patients with hidradenitis suppurativa. Dermatologic Surgery. 2000;**26**(7):638-643

[36] Deckers IE, Dahi Y, van der Zee HH, Prens EP. Hidradenitis suppurativa treated with wide excision and second intention healing: A meaningful local cure rate after 253 procedures. Journal of the European Academy of Dermatology and Venereology JEADV. 2018;**32**(3):459-462

[37] Manfredini M, Garbarino F, Bigi L, Pellacani G, Magnoni C. Hidradenitis suppurativa: Surgical and postsurgical management. Skin Appendage Disorders. 2020;**6**(4):195-201

[38] Humphries LS, Kueberuwa E, Beederman M, Gottlieb LJ. Wide excision and healing by secondary intent for the surgical treatment of hidradenitis suppurativa: A single-center experience. Journal of Plastic, Reconstructive & Aesthetic Surgery JPRAS. 2016;**69**(4):554-566

[39] Morgan WP, Harding KG, Hughes LE. A comparison of skin grafting and healing by granulation,

following axillary excision for hidradenitis suppurativa. Annals of the Royal College of Surgeons of England. 1983;**65**(4):235-236

[40] Pope ER. Mesh skin grafting. The Veterinary Clinics of North America. Small Animal Practice. 1990;**20**(1):177-187

[41] Morykwas MJ, Argenta LC, Shelton-Brown EI, McGuirt W. Vacuum-assisted closure: A new method for wound control and treatment: Animal studies and basic foundation. Annals of Plastic Surgery. 1997;**38**(6):553-562

[42] Chen E, Friedman HI. Management of regional hidradenitis suppurativa with vacuum-assisted closure and split thickness skin grafts. Annals of Plastic Surgery. 2011;**67**(4):397-401

[43] van Rappard DC, Mooij JE, Mekkes JR. Mild to moderate hidradenitis suppurativa treated with local excision and primary closure. Journal of the European Academy of Dermatology and Venereology JEADV. 2012;**26**(7):898-902

[44] Busnardo FF, Coltro PS, Olivan MV, Busnardo APV, Ferreira MC. The thoracodorsal artery perforator flap in the treatment of axillary hidradenitis suppurativa: Effect on preservation of arm abduction. Plastic and Reconstructive Surgery. 2011;**128**(4):949-953

[45] Geh JLC, Niranjan NS. Perforator-based fasciocutaneous island flaps for the reconstruction of axillary defects following excision of hidradenitis suppurativa. British Journal of Plastic Surgery. 2002;**55**(2):124-128

[46] Gibrila J, Chaput B, Boissière F, Atlan M, Fluieraru S, Bekara F. Radical treatment of hidradenitis suppurativa: Comparison of the use of the artificial dermis and pedicled perforator flaps. Annales de Chirurgie Plastique et Esthétique. 2019;**64**(3):224-236

[47] Ortiz CL, Castillo VL, Pilarte FS, Barraguer EL. Experience using the thoracodorsal artery perforator flap in axillary hidradentitis suppurativa cases. Aesthetic Plastic Surgery. 2010;**34**(6):785-792

[48] Rehman N, Kannan RY, Hassan S, Hart NB. Thoracodorsal artery perforator (TAP) type I V-Y advancement flap in axillary hidradenitis suppurativa. British Journal of Plastic Surgery. 2005;**58**(4):441-444

[49] Civelek B, Aksoy K, Bilgen E, İnal I, Sahin U, Çelebioğlu S. Reconstructive options in severe cases of hidradenitis suppurativa. Open Med. 2010;**5**(6):674-678

[50] Weigelt MA, Sanchez DP, Lev-Tov H. 20 - dressings and wound care supplies for hidradenitis suppurativa. In: Shi VY, Hsiao JL, Lowes MA, Hamzavi IH, editors. A Comprehensive Guide to Hidradenitis Suppurativa [Internet]. Philadelphia: Elsevier; 2022. pp. 201-207. Verfügbar unter: https://www.sciencedirect.com/science/article/pii/B9780323777247000206 [zitiert: Februar 18, 2024]

[51] Galazka AM. Beyond patient empowerment: Clinician-patient advocacy partnerships in wound healing. British Journal of Healthcare Management. 2019;**25**(6):1-6

[52] Ruan QZ, Chen AD, Singhal D, Lee BT, Fukudome EY. Surgical management of hidradenitis suppurativa: Procedural trends and risk factors. The Journal of Surgical Research. 2018;**229**:200-207

[53] Owens CD, Stoessel K. Surgical site infections: Epidemiology, microbiology

and prevention. The Journal of Hospital Infection. 2008;**70**(Suppl. 2):3-10

[54] Ritz JP, Runkel N, Haier J, Buhr HJ. Extent of surgery and recurrence rate of hidradenitis suppurativa. International Journal of Colorectal Disease. 1998;**13**(4):164-168

[55] Scholl L, Hessam S, Bergmann U, Bechara FG. Surgical treatment of sinus tracts and fistulas in perianal hidradenitis suppurativa. Journal of Cutaneous Medicine and Surgery. 2018;**22**(2):239-241

[56] Chapman S, Delgadillo D, Barber C, Khachemoune A. Cutaneous squamous cell carcinoma complicating hidradenitis suppurativa: A review of the prevalence, pathogenesis, and treatment of this dreaded complication. Acta Dermatovenerologica Alpina, Panonica et Adriatica. 2018;**27**(1):25-28

[57] Sachdeva M, Mufti A, Zaaroura H, Abduelmula A, Lansang RP, Bagit A. Squamous cell carcinoma arising within hidradenitis suppurativa: A literature review. International Journal of Dermatology. 2021;**60**(11):e459-e465

[58] Skorochod R, Margulis A, Adler N. Surgical management of hidradenitis suppurativa: Factors associated with postoperative complications and disease recurrence. Plastic and Reconstructive Surgery. Global Open. 2023;**11**(1):e4752

[59] Smith AD, Curtin GP, Allen NC, Fernandez-Penas P, Varey AH. Management of genital hidradenitis suppurativa and lymphoedema with the restoration of erectile function. The Australasian Journal of Dermatology. 2022;**63**(2):e184-e186

[60] Micieli R, Alavi A. Lymphedema in patients with hidradenitis suppurativa: A systematic review of published literature. International Journal of Dermatology. 2018;**57**(12):1471-1480

[61] Ly CL, Kataru RP, Mehrara BJ. Inflammatory manifestations of lymphedema. International Journal of Molecular Sciences. 2017;**18**(1):171

[62] Pacheco YD, García-Duque O, Fernández-Palacios J. Penile and scrotal lymphedema associated with hidradenitis suppurativa: Case report and review of surgical options. Cirugia y Cirujanos. 2019;**86**(1):77-80

[63] Yaman A, Borman P, Eşme P, Çalışkan E. Complex decongestive therapy in hidradenitis suppurativa-related genital lymphoedema: A case report. Journal of Wound Care. 2024;**33**(Suppl. 2a):xxviii-xxxi

[64] Musumeci ML, Scilletta A, Sorci F, Capuzzo G, Micali G. Genital lymphedema associated with hidradenitis suppurativa unresponsive to adalimumab treatment. JAAD Case Reports. 2019;**5**(4):326-328

[65] Corder B, Googe B, Velazquez A, Sullivan J, Arnold P. Surgical management of acquired buried penis and scrotal lymphedema: A retrospective review. Journal of Plastic, Reconstructive & Aesthetic Surgery JPRAS. 2023;**85**:18-23

[66] Rubaian NFB, Al Zamami HF, Almuhaidib SR, Al Breiki SH. Hidradenitis supparativa complicated by penoscrotal lymphedema and renal amyloidosis. Saudi Medical Journal. 2022;**43**(7):751-754

www.ingramcontent.com/pod-product-compliance
Lightning Source LLC
Chambersburg PA
CBHW081335190326
41458CB00018B/6009